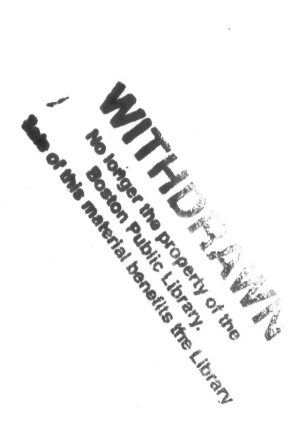

The
Checklist

The Checklist

WHAT YOU AND YOUR FAMILY
NEED TO KNOW TO PREVENT DISEASE
AND LIVE A LONG
AND HEALTHY LIFE

DR. MANNY ALVAREZ

An Imprint of HarperCollinsPublishers

THE CHECKLIST Copyright © 2007 by Manuel Alvarez. All rights reserved. Printed in the United States of America. No part of this book may be used or reproduced in any manner whatsoever without written permission except in the case of brief quotations embodied in critical articles and reviews. For information, address HarperCollins Publishers, 10 East 53rd Street, New York, NY 10022.

HarperCollins books may be purchased for educational, business, or sales promotional use. For information, please write: Special Markets Department, HarperCollins Publishers, 10 East 53rd Street, New York, NY 10022.

FIRST EDITION

Designed by Chris Welch

Library of Congress Cataloging-in-Publication Data
Alvarez, Manny.
    The checklist : what you and your family need to know to prevent disease and live a long and healthy life / Manny Alvarez.
        p. cm.
    Includes index.
    ISBN: 978-0-06-118878-7
    ISBN-10: 0-06-118878-6
    1. Health—Popular works.   2. Health promotion.   3. Medicine, Preventive.   I. Title.
RA776.A48 2007
613—dc22   2006050987

07 08 09 10 11 DIX/RRD 10 9 8 7 6 5 4 3 2 1

TO MY WIFE KATARINA AND CHILDREN REX, RYAN, AND OLIVIA

Acknowledgments

Many of the concepts in *The Checklist* are the culmination of all the great mentors I have had during my medical training—they have shaped my knowledge and given me tremendous love and respect for medicine. I am also grateful to all the wonderful patients I have met and treated; I have always learned something listening to their inquisitive questions. We have always been there for each other.

Thanks also to all my physician friends who provided me with feedback while writing this book, especially Dr. Michael Petriella, Dr. Julio Guerra, and Dr. Abdulla Al-Khan, as well as all the doctors and nurses of Hackensack University Medical Center.

I also wish to acknowledge my personal staff, Haydee Mato and Deborah Willems, for keeping up with my crazy schedule as I tried to complete this book. A special thanks to Leah Broida for her diligent research, Allyson Cacioli for her shorthand reporting, and Patrick Huyghe, a great science writer and friend, for his help with this book.

One person who deserves special credit is Roger Ailes, who provided me with a tremendous opportunity by signing me to do health stories at Fox News. His commitment to the American public is equal to none and for that and his friendship I will be eternally grateful. I also want to acknowledge all the wonderful and talented people at Fox News for mentoring me into the world of broadcasting.

I could not have worked with a better publishing house than Harper-Collins, whose professional staff made this process a wonderful experience. A big hug to the staff at Rayo Books, especially Ray Garcia, Rene Alegria, Melinda Moore, and Andrea Montejo.

Finally, I wish to express my gratitude to the family I love so much. I only wish my dad was still alive to see his son's new book, but I know he is watching. To my mother, sister, and nieces, please know that your love for me has kept me going. And, as always, I want to thank from the bottom of my heart my dear and lovely wife who has been a great support to me. I hope that this book will serve as an example for my children to grow up sharing the love and respect that I have for America.

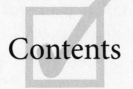

Contents

2

Life Is Beautiful
(The Second Decade: Ages 10 to 19)

Ah-choo ■ Asthma ■ Acne ■ Our supersized kids (obesity) ■ The best measure of weight (BMI) ■ Dental Health ■ Turning obesity on its head (bulimia) ■ Too thin (anorexia) ■ Depression ■ Substance Abuse ■ Cigarette smoking ■ Sexually Transmitted Diseases (STDs) ■ The kissing disease—mononucleosis ■ What's next

3

Welcome to the Real World
(The Third Decade: Ages 20 to 29)

Geek lifestyle ■ Debilitating headaches ■ Baby time—or not ■ Kicking the habit ■ Common skin conditions ■ Autoimmune but (thankfully) not automatic ■ The long winding road (gastrointestinal disorders) ■ Three decades down, the number left is up to you

4

Living Responsibly
(The Fourth Decade: Ages 30 to 39)

Nutrition ■ How to eat ■ Supplements ■ Skin health and cancer ■ A little gland with a big job ■ Bladder infections ■ Are you collecting stones? ■ Gynecological problems (for women only) ■ Cervical cancer ■ Infertility ■ Joints—the first to go ■ Rheumatoid arthritis ■ Fibromyalgia ■ Multiple sclerosis (MS) ■ Looking toward the next decade

8

The Beauty of Age
(The Eighth Decade and Beyond:
Ages 70 to 100) 259

Foreword

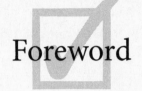

Perhaps you've seen him on TV? His name is Dr. Manny Alvarez, but everyone calls this warm and friendly physician of the airwaves Dr. Manny. For several years he has been the voice of health for Fox News, bringing the latest medical information to audiences all around the world.

Dr. Manny's experience as an academic leader in medicine has provided him with the tools necessary to easily connect with his patients and their families, giving them the information they can use and understand. Television has allowed him to share his knowledge and expand his care to an ever-growing audience hungry for health advice they can trust.

We know that preventative care is the key to a healthier future and Dr. Manny Alvarez is no stranger to this idea. While our book, *YOU: The Owner's Manual,* explained how our body works and what to do to keep it healthy and young, Dr. Manny's *The Checklist* is a complementary handbook that tells you what may go wrong with your body—decade by decade—and what you need to do in order to get to your next birthday feeling like time is not your enemy.

Our bodies need routine checkups to keep functioning properly and *The Checklist* tells you in an easy-to-read and well-organized fashion how to identify those problems that may arise over the course of your life. This is a book for the whole family, covering all ages, because, after all, when one member of our family gets sick, it affects us all.

So follow our advice, learn how your body works, and do what it takes to keep your body running healthily throughout your many birthdays.

Michael F. Roizen, M.D.

Mehmet C. Oz, M.D.

authors of *YOU: The Owner's Manual*

Introduction

Do health and medical facts and figures usually leave you puzzled? Are you overwhelmed with the amount of information you need to know to stay healthy? Does knowing how your body works still leave you wondering, "Well, okay, but what should I do? And when should I do it?" If so, then this is the right book for you.

Like most people you are probably getting your health news from television, magazines, newspapers, and the Internet. But there is often a disconnect between what we hear and read and how the latest medical discoveries apply to our age group. While certain diseases and health problems are a constant threat throughout our lives, many more are specific to a certain decade of life. A teenage boy isn't usually concerned with prostate disease, and it's rare for a sixty-five-year-old woman to worry about sexually transmitted diseases. It's quite obvious, isn't it? But what if you harnessed that knowledge—the knowledge that there is a time, a season, for every disease and health risk—and let it serve as a guide to living a healthy life?

What you would have is this book. *The Checklist* is a health maintenance book organized to help you identify and avoid the diseases and health risks you are most susceptible to during any given stage of your life.

The book will walk you through each phase of the aging process and help you take the right precautions, at the right time in your life, in order to avoid problems as you get older. Each chapter focuses on a particular living decade. Starting out with a preface that contains advice for the pregnant mother and unborn child, the book goes on to explore what diseases to look for and how to maintain solid health habits during your teens, your twenties, thirties, forties, up through your seventies.

As a person matures, each decade comes with certain risks that didn't exist in the previous decade of life. Each decade requires some very specific health knowledge that pertains to it specifically. Each decade's health plan must be tailor-made to fit a body as it matures, and sometimes this can differ between men and women, or boys and girls. If you act preventatively and proactively, based on the maintenance advice I present in this book, you should have a better chance of closing the door to future life-threatening diseases and other problems that may arise well into old age. I hope to bring clarity to confusing health concerns and help you understand your body as it ages.

You might choose to look at this book as a kind of manual of what to expect when you're in your teens, what to expect when you're in your twenties, etc. Of course, if you don't take the proper preventative steps for each decade, you will end up reading the book as a manual of what you may end up with when you are in your forties, or fifties, or whenever. Should you encounter one of the major problems of the decade you happen to be passing through, I will try to provide you with some advice on what to do and how to handle it.

Now I should add three caveats to fend off the critics who are already lining up at my door. First of all, I am well aware that many health issues may happen to you before or after the decade in which I have slotted them in this book. Because we are individuals, because we are all slightly different from one another, because things don't happen at the same time for everyone, there is an index at the back of the book that includes an alphabetical list of all the topics covered for easy lookup when you need it. Secondly, I will often use an analogy to the automobile in my discussions on health. I am well aware of the differences between an automobile and the human body. However, I do so for one simple reason: many people understand their car better than they do their own body, and if the analogy helps to clarify a point about human health, so much the better. Thirdly, I will not be able to cover every health issue that may happen to you in your lifetime. I won't be discussing statistically improbable diseases or rare medical conditions. If I mentioned every possible disease, every potential problem, for every age, this book would be too heavy to carry around, too expensive to buy, and, frankly, too imposing to be useful.

More than anything else I want this book to be a helpful resource for you. I want you to come to terms with the disconnect between the decade a disease or illness is likely to strike and when you should start thinking about its prevention. It's really too late to start keeping tabs on your cholesterol when you are sixty years old and already have heart disease. That's something you should start thinking about in your twenties. You need to exercise and watch your weight decades earlier. That's how the decades of your life tie in to one another and why early prevention is the key to good health. The preventive steps you ignore in one decade will catch up to you in another. It may not be the next decade, or the one after that, but sooner or later a poor diet or a destructive behavior will catch up with you.

I'm not saying prevention is easy; it's not. But it is rewarding. You'll feel better along the way, and when you get to your senior years, you'll be able to live a healthy and joyful life, instead of being hobbled with disease and medical problems. There will actually come a time when your age will cease to have any meaning other than chronological. If you're seventy years old, but your mind and body function like those of a fifty-year-old, why should anyone call you a seventy-year-old? If you've got a healthy heart, low cholesterol, and strong muscles; if you run, play golf or tennis, and your brain is sharp; if you're reading, writing, being productive, and enjoying life the way those who are twenty years younger than you are, what does being seventy years old really mean anymore? But in order to get there, in order to become truly ageless, you have to take care of yourself early on.

One of the things we don't do well in the United States with regard to health care is focus on preventive medicine. In many other countries medicine is all about prevention. But here, in the United States, we react to diseases only when they happen. We don't really try to prevent them from happening, and that's why the statistics for some diseases in this country are out of control. Let this book then be a tool for prevention.

True, some things are out of your control. If you're born with bad genes, you're born with bad genes. We are who we are. And, of course, nature can throw us a curve ball every once in a while and create unpredictable circumstances—cancer, trauma, genetic disease. All of this is out of your control. But everything else, or most everything else, is under your control. Invest in your body and your mind today, and you'll thank me and your doctor tomorrow. I guarantee it.

A Prenatal Preface

(for the Mother-to-Be)

**What? This isn't a decade. It's just nine months.
But are you prepared? The baby is "in the oven,"
and how well your little cake comes out
depends a lot on how ready you really are.
A proper prenatal environment ensures a
healthy first decade of life.**

Think Ahead

It's never too early to think about your health. In fact, the right time to think about it is *before* you are even born. Of course, you can't do that, and it's obviously too late for any of you reading this book, but it's not too late for the child you are planning to have. The prenatal health of a child is the parents' responsibility. What the mother and father do before they even *think* of having a child will help that future boy or girl get the right healthy start in life. So don't just show up pregnant at your doctor's office. It was unavoidable, you say? Really? Now let's get real: you need to have a physical *before* conceiving and discuss your desire to become pregnant with your physician.

The first topic of discussion will be your pregnancy history. If this is to be your first pregnancy, end of topic. If not, the doctor will ask you if you had any medical complications during prior pregnancies, and he will want to hear all about it, as the same complications are likely to arise again in your next pregnancy. For instance, if you had diabetes in your last pregnancy, you could have diabetes again. If you had preterm labor in your last pregnancy, you run the risk of preterm labor again. It's never absolutely guaranteed to be a rerun, but it's a good bet. It's good to know what you're up against in advance.

If this is going to be your first pregnancy, the doctor will want to know about your overall health. Have you had kidney disease, heart disease, or liver disease? These three organs are particularly important because they do double duty when you're pregnant. Your whole body chemistry, your whole physiology, goes into overdrive. Your body is not working only for you but for your baby as well. Typically, if anything is to go wrong during pregnancy, these are the organs we'll have to worry about.

The doctor will also want to know if you have allergies to any medication. During pregnancy you might receive antibiotics such as penicillin or penicillin-like drugs, pain medications such as Tylenol, as well as some short-acting narcotics such as Demerol and morphine. If you have any allergies, it's important to let your doctor know because you want to avoid having a reaction that will put you or your baby at risk.

Are you a smoker? Smoking is the number-one problem in a pregnancy. If you're thinking of having a baby and you smoke, stop smoking *now*. This is the perfect time to quit because smoking is, quite simply, very bad for you and your future child. Smoking is the number-one cause of lung cancer; it can also lead to chronic bronchitis, heart disease, and emphysema when you get older.

Smoking during pregnancy is one of the main reasons for delivering premature babies and for having babies who are too small for their age. In the obstetrical world, we call it IUGR, intrauterine growth retardation. The problem is that the placenta—the organ that serves as the interface between mother and child—is unable to filter out all the nicotine molecules, causing small vessel disease, which results in a small baby and perhaps preterm labor. So if you smoke, this is the time to quit.

Family history is, of course, very important. The doctor will want to know a little about your family pedigree. This applies to the two of you, both the mother and the father. Do either one of you have any family history of genetic diseases? Common genetic diseases include mental retardation, Down's syndrome, and cystic fibrosis, among others. Your child will be susceptible to different genetic diseases

Say No to Alcohol

Most women today are aware that drinking during pregnancy can cause physical and mental birth defects, but many do not realize that even light drinking may harm the fetus as well. If you're having a drink, baby is, too. Each year more than a thousand children are born in the United States with fetal alcohol syndrome, the most common cause of mental retardation in this country, and tens of thousands more are born with some degree of alcohol-related impairment. While the occasional drink a woman takes before she realizes she is pregnant is unlikely to harm her baby, mothers who are nursing should continue to abstain from alcohol. Alcohol is simply not acceptable during pregnancy and should always be discouraged. Don't take a chance with your baby's future.

depending on your ethnic background. If you're Jewish, for example, you're susceptible to diseases like Tay-Sachs (a fatal inherited disease of the central nervous system) and Bloom's syndrome (a disease that predisposes an individual to cancer and infections). If you're Greek, Italian, or of Mediterranean descent, one worry is the possibility of Mediterranean anemia (a shortage of the oxygen-carrying component of the blood). Work with your doctor to discover what particular diseases have affected members of your family in the past.

The obstetrician will also do a physical on the mother-to-be, checking blood pressure and weight and doing a blood test to see if she is anemic. The doctor will probably prescribe prenatal vitamins as well. Vitamins are important, especially folic acid. You want to make sure you're taking folic acid before you get pregnant to minimize the chance of neural tube defects such as spina bifida. The newest prenatal vitamins incorporate omega-3 fatty acids as a way to improve fetal brain development. The mother's weight and diet are extremely important, too. If you are overweight before you get pregnant, you should try to lose some weight. Losing weight before pregnancy improves not only your chance of conceiving, but also your chance of experiencing a normal childbirth. A healthy diet will help prepare the mother's body for bearing a child.

> ## What's a Good Source of Folic Acid?
>
> Breads and cereals, as well as eggs and liver, are good sources of folic acid. So are spinach, asparagus, orange juice, broccoli, corn, beets, celery, raspberries, cauliflower, tomato juice, green beans, strawberries, and other fruits and vegetables. Lentils, black beans, great northern beans, pinto beans, split peas, and peanuts also contain folic acid.

Nine Months and Counting

Once you are pregnant, your obstetrician will want to run some important laboratory tests. The standard laboratory tests are for anemia, hepatitis, rubella, and HIV. Some doctors will also test for sickle cell anemia, cystic fibrosis, and toxoplasmosis, a single-celled parasite that could cause serious problems during pregnancy. You will also get a *dating ultrasound* at this time, which will take the overall crown/rump measurement of the baby and help predict a more accurate delivery date.

Recently doctors have been focusing on early fetal development and the benefits of early screening. So at about twelve weeks of pregnancy you may get a new ultrasound scan called a *nuchal translucency* (NT) test and simple blood test, PAPP-A (pregnancy-associated plasma protein-A) and free beta-hCG. These tests are used to determine your risk of having a baby with Down's syndrome, which encompasses a number of chromosomal abnormalities. The most common is trisomy 21, which means that the egg has three 21st chromosomes instead of the normal two, resulting in a condition that may cause serious learning difficulties as well as physical disabilities. Other chromosomal disorders include trisomy 18 and trisomy 13. Of the genetic diseases found to date, these are the most common. Though the NT test offers an early accurate assessment of the risks of Down syndrome, other doctors opt for a test that has long been regarded as the "gold standard" test for Down's syndrome, the alpha fetal protein test, or AFP, at sixteen weeks. The AFP is a blood test that indirectly also helps identify babies at risk for Down syndrome and trisomy 18, as well as neural tube defects.

Depending on the results of these tests, your age, or your previous medical history, your obstetrician may offer an amniocentesis or even a CVS (chorionic villus sampling). Both of these tests are invasive, meaning that they require inserting a needle into the uterus to extract either amniotic fluid or a very small piece of placental tissue. They both provide very specific results on the genetic status of your newborn. A typical result will be 46XX, which is a normal female, or 46XY, which is a normal male, because the norm is to have 46 chromosomes in 23 pairs. But in the case of Down's syndrome or trisomy 21 the result would be 47XX, indicating three sets of chromosome 21.

Between the nineteenth and twentieth week you will get your first level-two ultrasound. The famous level-two ultrasound, or, as they like to call it, the targeted ultrasound, will detail the size of the baby by measuring all its bones: head, arms, forearms, legs, and abdomen. It also takes a look at the baby's internal structure, its brain anatomy, chest anatomy, abdominal anatomy, and the overall fetal environment, including where the placenta is located and how much fluid you have in the uterus. This anatomical survey can help identify problems that amniocentesis cannot rule out.

Ask Dr. Manny

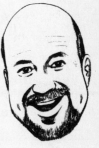

SEX DURING PREGNANCY

The key to intercourse during pregnancy is to keep it normal—with a few caveats.

IS IT SAFE TO HAVE SEX WHEN YOU'RE PREGNANT?

Usually, yes. In fact, many expectant mothers find that their sexual desire is enhanced at different stages of their pregnancy. Of course, as they get bigger, a lot of women find that sex becomes uncomfortable. After four or five months of pregnancy, it's very difficult for a woman to lie on her back, so side-to-side intercourse or the woman-on-top position may be preferable to the missionary position. It's important to keep the lines of communication open between you and your partner on this subject, and with your obstetrician as well.

Intercourse during pregnancy may not be recommended under certain medical conditions, however. Your obstetrician may be concerned if you've had a history of miscarriage or preterm labor, *placenta previa* (when the placenta is implanted in the lower segment of the uterus), *incompetent cervix* (when the cervix is weakened and dilated, which can lead to prematurity), multiple pregnancy (twins, triplets, etc.), cramping after intercourse, unexplained vaginal bleeding, or a leakage of amniotic fluids. Of course, if you don't know the sexual history of your partner, sexually transmitted infections are of concern as well.

(continued on next page)

(**Ask Dr. Manny** continued from previous page)

CAN SEX HARM THE BABY?

No, not directly. The baby is protected by the uterus and the membranes. There's also a very thick mucous plug inside the cervix that guards against infections.

WHEN CAN YOU RESUME SEX AFTER DELIVERY?

You should wait until your postpartum checkup with your gynecologist before you resume intercourse. But if you feel a loss of sexual drive after childbirth, don't worry; it's perfectly normal and probably temporary. This is most likely due to the hormonal changes that occur in childbirth, as well as to the general trauma of childbirth to the vaginal canal. The stress and exhaustion that come from dealing with a newborn baby also play a major role in some women not wanting to have intercourse at this time of their lives.

The Three Major Prenatal Problems

The vast majority of all medical complications during pregnancy fall into one of the following three categories: hypertension, diabetes, and premature labor. Let's take a closer look at each one of these.

When Normal Is Too High

You are now well into your pregnancy, but every obstetrical visit will still include a measure of your blood pressure. Blood pressure is the force of the blood pushing against the walls of your arteries, which are the blood vessels that carry oxygen-rich blood away from the heart to all parts of your body. When the pressure on the arteries becomes too high, it's called *hypertension*. About 5 percent of women have hypertension before they become pregnant. This is called *chronic hypertension*. Another 5 percent or so develop hypertension during pregnancy. This is called *gestational hypertension.* Oddly enough, a normal person's blood pressure reading may actually signal hypertension during pregnancy. Why? Because all the natural hormones your body pumps out during pregnancy end up dilating your blood vessels, which should produce a blood pressure at the low end of the normal range. So if yours is at the upper end of the normal range, your blood pressure is, relatively speaking, too high.

Most reasons for hypertension during pregnancy are unknown. Certainly, if you have a history of hypertension, pregnancy could just exacerbate the condition. But obesity and stress can also have a compound effect on your blood pressure during pregnancy. Hypertension is a particularly worrisome issue during pregnancy because it can constrict the blood vessels in the uterus, which supply the fetus with the necessary oxygen and nutrients. This can slow the fetal growth and result in a low birth weight. Hypertension also increases the risk of a *preterm delivery,* that is, a delivery that occurs before your thirty-seventh week. Both low birth weight and prematurity not only increase the risk of health problems for newborns but may result in learning problems and the delayed development of motor skills later on.

The treatment for hypertension during pregnancy is limited. A doctor will generally recommend that a pregnant woman with early or mild hypertension cut back on her activities and avoid strenuous exercise, while more serious cases require hospitalization.

Dangerously High

Excessively high blood pressure during pregnancy can cause many problems. One is a condition called *placental abruption.* This is a premature separation of the placenta from the uterine wall, a condition that would typically cause vaginal bleeding and uterine contractions. If the abruption jeopardizes your health or your baby's health, you'll need to have an immediate delivery. Another high blood pressure problem is a rare but life-threatening condition called preclampsia. This occurs when high blood pressure is accompanied by protein in the urine. The mechanisms leading to precalmpsia are not clear, but this condition can quickly worsen and jeopardize the life of both mother and baby. If the fetus is less than thirty-four weeks old, a drug called a corticosteroid may be administered to help speed up the maturity of the fetal lungs. On the other hand, if it occurs after the thirty-seventh week, the physician may recommend inducing delivery. The only real cure for preclampsia is delivery. Receiving regular prenatal care allows your doctor to deal with the problems that might arise from hypertension early on.

Not So Sweet

When you're pregnant, it's breakfast, lunch, and dinner for two every day for nine months. Your body provides your baby with its *only* source of nourishment. And that source of nourishment is also your own body's source of nourishment—the glucose that results from the breakdown of carbohydrates in your body. This glucose is delivered from your bloodstream to the muscles and other cells that need this fuel through a hormone called *insulin*. When your body fails to produce enough insulin, the glucose builds up in your body, which can possibly result in diabetes. There is never a good time to have diabetes, but there is no worse time than during pregnancy, as it puts two of you at risk.

During pregnancy, your body delivers glucose to the baby through the placenta, a temporary organ that also provides the baby with oxygen and serves to pass out the baby's waste. (After birth the placenta is called the *afterbirth*.) For its limited existence, this organ has a tremendous workload, including producing hormones that assist in the baby's development. Trouble is, the natural hormones of pregnancy, which are designed to break down your fat cells into glucose, may create more glucose in your system than your body can adequately metabolize. The result is *gestational diabetes*. If, on top of that, your diet is high in sugar by-products—in other words, if you are taking in large amounts of carbohydrates and sugar through candies and cakes—this second source of glucose coming in from the outside may put you over the threshold.

Pregnancy affects the blood glucose levels in all women, so at twenty-eight weeks you're going to be screened for diabetes. Diabetes is a very common problem in pregnancy and some women who are nearly diabetic when they get pregnant will go right over the edge and experience this glucose intolerance, and the inability to process all the glucose in their system. The problem with diabetes in pregnancy is that it often leads to the birth of large babies, because the excess glucose goes to the baby directly. In other words, if mommy has high sugar, the baby has high sugar.

And it affects you as an individual—by frequent urination, weight gain, and restricted movements—the same way it affects the baby in utero. The baby gets excessively large and urinates frequently, changing the composition of the fetal fluid, which may even put the baby at risk of death. The other problem with large babies is that they tend to suffer more trauma during vaginal delivery—broken collarbones, for instance, or injury to the nerves in the neck called the *brachial plexus*. Large babies also have a very difficult time as newborns because they're so overweight that they may suffer from a variety of metabolic disorders.

To test for diabetes, the physician will administer a challenge test. You'll be asked to drink a glucose solution in a soda-style liquid. After an hour, your glucose level will be measured. If the reading is too high, which occurs about 20 percent of the time, your doctor will have you come back for a glucose tolerance test. The good news is that most women whose challenge test comes back high don't turn out to have gestational diabetes after this follow-up test. But if your blood sugar level is still high, the doctor will put you on a diabetic diet based on complex carbohydrates, proteins, and vegetables. You will then need to monitor your sugar on a daily basis. If it continues to be elevated after a week or two, then you might need to start taking medication, such as insulin or oral hypoglycemic agents. The aim, whether by diet or medication, is to bring down your blood sugar to a level that will hopefully not interfere with your pregnancy.

Ready or Not

Every day one in eight babies born in the United States arrives sooner than expected. Premature birth is another common problem of pregnancy, and it can happen to anyone. By definition, a premature birth is one that occurs before the thirty-seventh week of pregnancy. The average size of a baby at thirty-seven weeks is about five pounds. However, since the field of neonatology has improved dramatically in the last couple of decades, a baby born healthy at thirty-five weeks has an overwhelmingly good prognosis for long-term survival. So more and more these days the definition of preterm labor has to do with how early in the pregnancy it occurs relative to the health of the baby. Prematurity can grossly compromise a child's quality of life and put the child at risk for deafness, cerebral palsy, and blindness.

Just what causes premature birth, no one knows for certain. Some research suggests that one of the main contributing factors to preterm labor is infection. Though such infections must be occurring quietly, without showing any symptoms, the bacteria in the cervix must be causing an inflammation, and the by-products of that inflammation are chemicals that can induce preterm labor. In other cases, women who have no infection may have a relatively weak uterus, or their cervix just doesn't have the integrity to hold the pregnancy as the baby gets bigger, thus allowing the cervix to open up early on. Still other women may have anatomical deformities of the uterus that again may put them at risk for preterm labor. Another probable cause of premature birth is stress. And as everyone knows who has been through it, stress is certainly a big factor in pregnancy.

The typical signs of premature labor are lower back pain, vaginal bleeding, excessive vaginal discharge, and premature contractions. Preterm labor is treated by such medications as magnesium sulfate, terbutaline sulfate, and antibiotics—all of which aim, though with limited results, to stop those contractions. Women in premature labor are often given steroids. Steroids? Yes, not all steroids are bad for you. When used appropriately in the right circumstances and under a doctor's supervision, steroids are a wonder. They are given to women experiencing premature labor in order to literally pump the baby up. Like turning up the heat on the stove to boil the potatoes a little quicker, the steroids help mature the baby's physiology more quickly so that he or she—however small—has a better chance of survival at birth.

Five Illnesses to Avoid During Pregnancy

If the mother-to-be is exposed to any of the following, see your doctor immediately.

- Fifth disease is caused by the parovirus and can cause anemia in your baby. If you get fifth disease early in your pregnancy, you could have a miscarriage.
- Chickenpox is caused by the varicella virus and can cause birth defects.
- Rubella, or German measles, is now rare, but it used to be a common cause of birth defects. Pregnant women should be tested to see if they're immune to rubella.
- Cytomegalovirus (CMV) is a common infection that can be passed from the mother to the baby, and it can cause birth defects. It doesn't produce symptoms, and there is no way to treat it. Those most at risk are those who work in day-care or health-care settings. Wash your hands after handling diapers and avoid nuzzling the babies.
- Toxoplasmosis is an infection caused by parasites from raw or uncooked infected meat or from contact with the feces of a cat. It can result in stillbirth, or death shortly after birth, and can cause mental- or motor-developmental delays, cerebral palsy, epilepsy and visual impairments, including sometimes blindness. Cook meats well, wash or peel fruits and vegetables, wear gloves while gardening, and have others change the kitty litter.

Fasten Your Seat Belts

Toward the third trimester you're going to start planning what I like to call "the landing of the aircraft." Fasten your seat belts, put your seat back in the upright position, remove all the glasses and utensils because we're ready to land. This really means assessing how you're going to deliver, whether vaginally or by cesarean section (C section), and, of course, running some tests on the fluid around the baby and the baby's breathing to determine just how strong the baby is for birth.

Finally, the big moment nears. When the baby's head drops down into the pelvis, it pushes against the cervix, the lower part of the uterus that opens into the vagina. This causes the cervix to relax, stretch out, and finally open to prepare for the passage of the baby through the vagina, or birth canal. When this occurs, most women in labor are sent to the hospital for labor and delivery. There, a vaginal examination will measure the *dilation,* or opening, of the cervix. Typically the cervix of a woman in active labor is dilated four centimeters, and she is having contractions every three to four minutes. If this is your first baby, you will usually dilate 1 to 1.2 centimeters an hour. If you have had other vaginal deliveries, typically you dilate 1.5 centimeters an hour. If you don't think three-tenths of a centimeter is much of a difference, you've never given birth. The faster you dilate, the quicker it's all over.

Sometimes complications occur during pregnancy, or during the birth itself, and a procedure called a *cesarean section* becomes necessary. If, in the course of vaginal labor, the baby seems not to be descending adequately, or the mother's cervix isn't dilated enough, or the baby is not tolerating the birth process, which is indicated by a dipping or slowing down of its heart rate, then your obstetrician may choose to do a cesarean section. Many times cesareans are performed without any labor if the baby is not properly oriented for birth (called *malpresentation*), if there are medical complications of pregnancy, or if a baby is premature.

If the delivery is progressing normally, once you get to full dilatation, ten centimeters, you're ready to push. Pushing is a very important phase of the vaginal delivery because it brings the head down as well as rotates the head into position for a successful vaginal birth. This is where coaching becomes important, where the father, or significant other, gets involved. The days of dads smoking a cigar in the waiting room are history. Delivery is now a family affair, as it should be. The coach provides the mother-to-be with the mental stamina to push through the course of the often-difficult two or three hours that follow. But no matter how many times you've rehearsed for this moment in the

The C-Section

About 29 percent of births in the United States are C-sections. A C-section is major surgery that involves the delivery of the baby via a surgical incision made through the abdominal wall and uterus, and thus may involve such complications as bleeding and infection. Certainly a cesarean birth has a longer recovery period than a vaginal birth, but most obstetrical centers are very well versed in this type of surgery. It can be performed within minutes of the obstetrician's decision to do one. It takes about five minutes from the time the initial incision is made until the baby is born, and another thirty minutes or so to complete the surgery.

And if you're wondering why it's called a cesarean, it's widely believed that Julius Caesar was born that way (though that's probably not true).

birthing classes you've taken together beginning since the twenty-eighth week of your pregnancy, you'll both find the moment a challenge. It's a kind of marathon run with the most incredible prize for all participants at the finish line.

Test Checklist for this Decade

	Blood tests
	Pap smear
	Urine test
	Ultrasound
	Amniocentesis (optional)
	Nonstress test (if high-risk pregnancy)

The Most Important Years of Your Life

(The First Decade: Ages 0 to 9)

1

This is the carefree decade,
though you won't realize that for another
decade or more. You will be completely taken
care of by your parents. All you have to do
is play and enjoy life. There are no worries for
you; your parents will be doing plenty of that.
These are the most important years of your life.
What your parents do for you now establishes
the foundation on which your future mental
and physical health rests.

Every time I deliver a baby, the beauty of the newborn amazes me. I always wonder if they are already longing for the days and months of warmth in their mother's body. They are so beautiful and perfect. Yet from the moment a child is born we start counting the days and the many firsts that accompany them: the first visit to the pediatrician, the first vaccination, the first day of preschool . . . wait, let's back up a moment.

A minute after birth there is life's first test, administered by the pediatrician or nurse in the birthing room. The Apgar test, as it's called, is a quick evaluation of the newborn's physical condition that determines if the baby needs emergency care. If the baby has good Apgar scores and looks fine, the baby is handed over to the mother so that the very important bonding process can begin immediately. (See "Welcome to the World," page 20.)

Bonding is one of the most beautiful moments of human life. Bonding reestablishes a physical attachment to the mother, after the physical detachment from the womb at birth, and forges the emotional and psychological attachments the child will need to thrive in the world. Bonding with the father is important as well. Fathers can bond with their children by holding them, helping them get to sleep, and giving them baths. A firm bond between the mother and child, and between the father and child, will boost the child's self-esteem, which in turn will affect how well the child does later in school and how he or she will build relationships with friends and react to stressful or new situations later in life.

Welcome to the World—Here Is Your First Test

The Apgar test was designed to quickly evaluate a newborn's physical condition. It is usually given to the baby twice, once at one minute after birth and again at five minutes after birth. Though named after anesthesiologist Virginia Apgar, who developed the test in 1952, it has also become an acronym for the test's five measures: **A**ctivity (muscle tone), **P**ulse (heart rate), **G**rimace (responsiveness), **A**ppearance (skin coloration), and **R**espiration (breathing). Each of the measures counts for two points, and the maximum score is ten, but, as in ice skating, a perfect ten is rare. If a baby gets a score of seven or more, he or she is considered to be in good health. A lower score simply means that the baby needs immediate care, such as a suctioning of the airways or a little oxygen to help him or her breathe. The Apgar test is by no means a measure of the baby's long-term health.

APGAR Score

	2	1	0
ACTIVITY	Active, spontaneous movement	Arms and legs flexed with little movement	No movement
HEART RATE	Normal pulse (above 100 beats per minute)	Pulse is below 100 beats per minute	No pulse
GRIMACE	Pulls away, sneezes, or coughs with stimulation	Stimulation only produces facial movement	No response to stimulation
APPEARANCE	Hands and feet are normal color all over	Normal facial color but hands and feet are bluish	Bluish gray or pale all over
BREATHING	Normal rate and effort	Slow or irregular breathing	No breathing

To Breast-feed or Not?

Now is the perfect time to begin breast-feeding. By continuing to nourish your child with your own body as you have done for nine months, you will ensure a healthy future not only for your child but for yourself as well. This may sound like a big promise, but it's one that delivers. Breast-feeding is very important because it significantly reduces the risk for all sorts of allergies and improves the baby's health as well as the mother's. Not only does it improve her metabolism, it definitely has some long-term protective benefits for the breast health of the mother. Some studies have shown that women who have breast-fed a child have lower breast cancer rates.

Typically, breast-feeding is recommended for anywhere between six months to a year. The longer you do it, the better. But most women cannot breast-feed after six months, and doing it even for just a month or two is fine, too. A little bit is better than nothing at all.

Many mothers, however, will choose to use baby formula instead. Most formulas today are nutritionally balanced with the right minerals, vitamins, and iron. While formula is effective, it does lack immunoglobulins, the antibodies found in breast milk that protect the child's ears, nose, throat, and gastrointestinal tract from viral and bacterial infections. (The mother's milk is said to be environmentally specific, meaning that her milk specifically protects her infant from the organisms to which the infant is most likely to be exposed.) There are many kinds of formulas, of course. For instance, soy-based formulas are especially made for babies who become intolerant to regular formula. Speak to your pediatrician about finding the right formula for your baby.

Cord Blood

Some mothers are now storing their infant's umbilical cord blood upon delivery, and you might want to think about doing so as well.

First, a quick explanation of what umbilical cord blood is. When a baby is born, the umbilical cord is clamped and cut to separate the infant from the mother. The portion of the cord that is attached to the placenta is removed from the mother's body and is usually discarded. Inside the cord are blood vessels that contain a good half cup of blood that belongs to the baby. That blood contains many stem cells. Our body uses stem cells as a way of repairing itself. Many parents are now choosing to collect and store that umbilical cord blood in case those cells are needed for their child somewhere down the line. It's like backing up files on your computer in case your hard drive crashes.

But how can a human "hard drive" crash? Let's take, as an example, the case of childhood leukemia, a cancer of the blood system. (See "Childhood Leukemia," page 22.) Many children who develop leukemia get effective treatments, but those treatments eliminate not only the cancer cells but some of the healthy cells as well. The child's "hard drive" gets erased, so to speak.

Typically, patients need to replenish their system with new cells—usually from another source, like bone marrow from a compatible donor. But finding a compatible donor is not an easy task. So more and more cancer centers are now relying on umbilical cord blood for several reasons: better grafting, perfect compatibility, and a reliable source—yourself! Almost all cancer specialists prefer a perfect match.

Imagine having your own cells to regenerate your system back to normal. This is one of the concepts behind storing a child's umbilical cord blood.

Childhood Leukemia

More than one-quarter of all cancers in children under the age of nineteen are leukemia. (Also see "Cancer of the Blood," page 207.) The most common form of leukemia in children is acute lymphocytic leukemia (ALL). The incidence of this leukemia among children one to four years of age is more than ten times greater than the rate for young adults ages twenty to twenty-four. The rates of leukemia are substantially higher among white children than in black children, but Hispanic children have the highest rates of all. There are about thirty-five hundred cases of leukemia in children a year, which results in about four hundred deaths a year. But the death rate for children up to fourteen years of age with leukemia in the United States has declined 60 percent over the past three decades. Although it's a long and difficult process, thanks to chemotherapy most children with ALL can now be cured.

Perhaps someday in the future we will be able to use one of those stored umbilical cord blood cells from a child with diabetes, for example, to grow a new pancreas for the child. That's the promise of an exciting new field called *regenerative medicine* that we'll be hearing much about in the future.

Beyond the "Baby Blues"

It's common for women to experience the "baby" or maternity blues after their pregnancy. These blues can last anywhere from a few hours to several days and include tears, headaches, irritability, sleeplessness, and a lack of concentration.

But 10 to 15 percent of women experience a serious depression during or after delivery. This is known as *postpartum depression* or PPD. It's widely believed that postpartum depression is due to hormonal changes after childbirth or to lifestyle changes brought about by the stress of pregnancy. The symptoms and treatment for PPD are the same as for any major depression (see "Depression," page 79).

The important thing about PPD is that it interferes with the mother's ability to nurture the newborn child. Partners and family members need to be aware of this potential problem so that it can be diagnosed and treated in time. Mothers should be encouraged to speak up about their feelings, and they should seek counseling and medical intervention if needed. Partners need to be supportive of their spouses if and when this problem arises. Some states have taken a leadership role on the issue: by law, New Jersey, for example, now requires doctors to educate expectant mothers and their families about postpartum depression and to screen new mothers for the condition.

To Cut or Not?

Many parents who have a boy ask themselves whether they should circumcise their baby or not. Circumcision goes back at least as far as Abraham's covenant with God, so this procedure has been around for ages.

But modern data does not support the *medical* need for circumcision. The position of the American Academy of Pediatrics (AAP), which has regularly reexamined the issue, is that newborn circumcision has potential medical benefits as well as risks. It has long been assumed that circumcision assures better penile hygiene, but the AAP found little evidence to support the association between circumcision and easily maintained good penile hygiene. Nonetheless, they did find that there is an increased risk of urinary tract infections in uncircumcised males. When it comes to the relationship between circumcision and sexually transmitted diseases, the AAP found the studies "complex and conflicting." But they did cite studies suggesting that circumcised males may be less at risk for syphilis than uncircumcised males, and they note that there is a substantial body of evidence linking noncircumcised men with risk for HIV infection. The AAP also found that the risk of penile cancer in an uncircumcised man is three times more likely than in a circumcised man, though penile cancer is rare in the United States, just one in one hundred thousand males has it. As for complications with newborn circumcision, they certainly can occur, noted the AAP, but the rate is just a few tenths of a percent of those who are circumcised, and those that do occur involve bleeding and infection and are usually minor.

Since circumcision is no longer regarded as a medical necessity, most circumcisions today are performed for either religious or cultural reasons. If the grandfather was circumcised, and the father was circumcised, the son is likely to be circumcised as well; it's a family tradition. Whites are more likely to be circumcised than blacks, and Hispanics even less so than blacks. Some religions favor circumcision; Jews, for example, regard circumcision as a religious ritual.

Circumcisions are usually done within twenty-four hours of the baby's birth and in the hospital, typically by the obstetrician. After applying a local anesthetic, the foreskin is retracted, and one centimeter or so of the foreskin is removed. The procedure is standard and done every day.

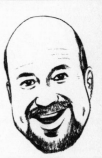

Ask Dr. Manny

TO PIERCE OR NOT?

"Dr. Manny, my little girl is two months old, and I really want to have her ears pierced, but my mother-in-law says it's not safe. Is this true?"

More and more parents are having their little girl's ears pierced soon after birth. But two months old may be a little too soon. Most pediatricians recommend that parents wait at least until their baby has had her second set of tetanus shots at the age of four months to avoid the risk of infection. And if you do have your infant's ears pierced, be sure to keep the earrings in a sterile environment, and use straight posts rather than hoop earrings to avoid having the infant's earlobe ripped off accidentally. You should also be aware that earrings can pose a choking hazard to the baby. So those are things you should think about.

On the other hand, some parents intending to have their child's ears pierced may be waiting too long. Ears should probably be pierced before the age of eleven to avoid keloids, those overgrowths of scar tissue that follow skin injuries, with ear piercing being a primary example. One study showed that those who had piercing at eleven years of age or older were more likely to develop keloids than were those who had piercings done before that age.

SIDS

The leading cause of death in otherwise healthy babies more than a month old is SIDS, or sudden infant death syndrome. It occurs in about fifty of every one hundred thousand births in the United States. SIDS applies to any infant whose death is sudden and unexplained. Usually the infant is found dead after having been put to sleep, and a subsequent autopsy finds absolutely nothing wrong with the baby. For the parents, it is the most horrific of experiences.

No one knows what causes SIDS but there are several risk factors associated with it. Babies who are born prematurely are at increased risk for SIDS; so are those who are exposed to tobacco smoke. Laying an infant to sleep on his or her stomach also increases the risk, as does excess bedding, a soft sleep surface, and the presence of stuffed animals.

There is no surefire way to prevent SIDS, but in light of these known risks, parents can take several precautions to reduce its likelihood. Don't smoke during pregnancy or anywhere in the house afterward. Don't overstuff the baby's crib with blankets or stuffed animals; small infants have little control of their heads and may smother themselves in their bedding. When you choose a crib, make sure it's a standard, federally recommended crib with a firm surface. Also, put your baby to sleep on his back, never his stomach. And above all, don't let the baby sleep with you in your own bed. More and more evidence suggests that parents, especially overweight ones, may inadvertently smother their babies when they're sleeping with their child, leading to SIDS. Finally, breast-feeding and pacifiers may also reduce the risk of SIDS. One recent study showed that breast-fed infants are five times less likely to have SIDS as

Seven Quick Tips to Avoid SIDs

To reduce the risk of SIDs, keep these dos and don'ts in mind:

- Don't smoke in the house
- Don't sleep with your baby
- Do choose a crib with a firm surface
- Do keep blankets and stuffed animals to a minimum
- Do place baby on his or her back to sleep
- Do breast-feed if you can
- Do use a pacifier

infants who have been formula fed. Another recent study has noted that the use of pacifiers is associated with a 90 percent decrease in the risk of SIDS.

Food Allergies

Nutrition is very important. It should be foremost on a parent's mind right from the beginning because if you teach your child how to eat properly in early childhood, you'll be able to avoid childhood obesity, now a serious epidemic in the United States. It also is important to teach an infant how to eat properly because one of the things you want to prevent is a food allergy.

A food allergy is a hypersensitivity, an abnormal response to food triggered by the immune system. About 6 percent of children under the age of three will have a food allergy. The most common ones are caused by milk, eggs, wheat, and peanuts. Peanut allergies can be so severe and hit so fast that if an allergic person encounters a peanut it could mean almost instant death. Cases of peanut allergies have doubled over the past ten years. At the moment the only available treatment is avoidance. But eliminating a specific food is easier said than done. Breast-feeding moms should even avoid putting moisturizers that contain peanut oil on their breasts and nipples. The protein associated with egg allergies is usually albumin, which may be present in pasta and marshmallows. To avoid problems, make sure you read all food and product labels carefully.

Many food allergies can be prevented with a proper nutrition schedule. All you have to do is follow a few simple rules. No solids until the baby is six months old, with the exception of cereals, which should be introduced between four and six months in order to minimize the risk of a wheat allergy. No whole milk or dairy products until the age of one. No eggs until the age of two. And no peanuts, or nuts at all for that matter, until the age of three.

Following these few simple rules will not guarantee that your child will grow up allergy-free, however. If you come from an allergic family, you are likely to be allergic, too. But minimizing the premature introduction of these foods will allow your child's immune system to adapt and develop in such a way that it can tolerate these foods and not regard them as poisons. That is what an allergic reaction is: it's your immune system reacting to something it thinks is not good for itself by releasing histamines. These histamines produce all the effects of an allergy—the rash, the runny nose—and if it's severe enough, the anaphylactic shock, which is a swelling of the tongue and difficulty breathing; many times—if not treated immediately—anaphylactic shock can lead to death. The good news for

Ask Dr. Manny

VITAMINS AND SUPPLEMENTS FOR KIDS

"Dr. Manny, I've got an eight-year-old son and a six-year-old daughter. My son will eat anything I give him, but my daughter is the definition of picky—she'll eat only pasta, pizza, and chicken. Should I be giving her vitamins? What about other supplements?"

If your son is eating well-balanced meals, he does not need vitamins. But your daughter, like so many young kids, isn't eating properly and should be given vitamins. A child can start taking vitamins at the age of three, and many kids today need them. Did you know that 20 to 25 percent of kids are calcium deficient? They just don't drink as much milk these days as kids used to, and they need the extra calcium. And how many young kids are eating their vegetables? Not many. That makes the B complex vitamins a good idea for them, too. And when they are on antibiotics, they should be taking acidophilus, the good bacteria for the gut that can be found in yogurt as well as in pill form, but always check with your pediatrician first. Acidophilus should be taken both during the antibiotic treatment and for two weeks afterward to repopulate your gut with the good bacteria that the antibiotic kills off along with the bad bacteria.

many food allergy sufferers is that time heals all; many people simply out-grow their allergies.

Loading the Virus Protection Program

If you have a computer, you know how important it is to install a program that protects it from computer viruses. Your immune system does a similar job against human viruses and bacteria. Essentially, it's a system of specialized cells and organs that protects you from outside threats such as viruses, bacteria, and other biological outsiders. Your immune system comes preloaded, but it's during the first decade of life that it learns which biological intrusions it needs to protect you against. What this means is, if you don't get exposed to many of the harmless biological threats in your environment during your first decade of life, that is, if you don't challenge your immune system early, you may pay the price with seasonal allergies and asthma in the second decade, and perhaps throughout the rest of your life as well.

What I'm talking about here are the dangers of overprotecting our children. Some of this overprotection has been institutionalized—it comes from the widespread use of antibiotics, vaccinations against various diseases, cleaner food and water, and better living conditions. But some parents may make this "problem" worse by keeping their kids at home in a "sterilized" environment: never taking them to the park, never letting them play in the sandbox, never letting them make mud pies, never letting them roll around in the grass, never letting them have a pet at home to play with, and keeping them away from any kids who may be sick. By underexposing our children to bacteria, certain viruses, and other minor threats in the environment, their immune systems will not develop the appropriate responses, and they may end up with seasonal allergies and other problems of an inexperienced immune system.

Studies show that if you have a pet when you're a kid, you are less likely to get asthma. The same applies to running and rolling around in the grass at the park when you are three years old; those who do tend to have fewer seasonal allergies later on. A little exposure is a good thing. Your kid's immune system will thank you later on. Well, not really, but you know what I mean.

Childproofing the Home

Having children keeps me on my toes. I am one of those parents who is always checking up on the kids—it drives my wife crazy! I have to admit this obsessive-compulsive behavior of mine could drive anyone crazy. But can you blame me? I have spent most of my adult life in hospitals, and one of the most heartbreaking things I see is when a child is rushed into the emergency room with an accidental overdose or poisoning.

Each year more than six thousand people die, and an estimated three hundred thousand suffer disabilities, as a result of unintentional poisoning. Not all of them are children, but children certainly are the most vulnerable. If you have children, one of the most fundamental things you must do is childproof your home. Of course, there is no such thing as a totally childproof home, but we have to try. Toddlers and young children are curious creatures, and as their mobility increases, their exposure to the potential dangers of a home will increase as well. They will climb anything, touch everything, and put anything that fits—or doesn't—into their mouths. Life can't be risk-free, but most household accidents can be prevented if you follow this checklist for household safety. Here are a few tips you can follow to make sure your home is as safe as possible for your child:

To Prevent Poisoning

Keep all medications—both prescription and nonprescription—as well as vitamins and supplements far from a child's reach. Don't leave any medications in your purse or pants pockets either; children may find them when searching for things to play with. And don't ever tell a child that a medication tastes like "candy." Keep household cleaning products, cosmetics and other toiletries, automotive and garden products, and other toxins in a high cabinet far from their reach. Don't leave alcoholic drinks and mouthwash, which contains alcohol, where children can reach them.

Two other types of poisoning should be guarded against: lead poisoning and carbon monoxide poisoning. If you live in a house that was built before 1978 (the year the use of lead paint was banned), the paint on the walls of your home may present a serious threat to the central nervous systems of your child. Lead toxicity in the blood can impair school performance and negatively affect cognitive functioning into young adulthood. The only solution is to move to a lead-free home, or to have the lead paint safely removed by certified lead contractors.

It is also important that you have a carbon monoxide monitor in the house. There are hundreds of fatalities due to carbon monoxide every year. It is *the* most toxic substance you'll come into contact with in your daily life, and it's not just caused by gas appliances. All fossil fuels, including oil, coal, and wood, are equally dangerous. The problem with carbon monoxide, of course, is that you can't smell it, see it, or taste it. It's fast-acting and deadly.

To Prevent Burns

Burns are among the most common of childhood accidents, so set the thermostat on your hot water heater to 120°F or lower. If you live in an apartment and have no control over the hot water temperature, install an antiscald device on your faucets. Don't use tablecloths or large place mats, as small children can—and will—pull on them, possibly overturning a hot drink or hot plate of food. Always turn pot and pan handles toward the back of the stove out of a child's reach. And even though it's mandatory in many cities and apartments today, always make sure you have a functioning fire alarm in the house.

To Prevent Strangulation

Tie up window blind cords so they are out of your child's reach. Cut cords so there is no loop at the bottom. Don't put necklaces or headbands on your baby, and never tie a pacifier around your baby's neck.

To Prevent Injuries from Firearms

Don't keep guns at home, and avoid exposing your children to households where guns are kept. Accidental shootings take the lives of 250 children aged fourteen and under in the United States each year. If you must keep a gun at home, store it in a securely locked case, out of a child's reach, and also keep the ammunition in a separate locked location.

To Prevent Injuries from Falls

Install safety bars on high windows, or close and lock such windows. Apply nonskid strips to the bottoms of bathtubs.

To Prevent Electric Shock

Cover all unused electrical outlets, which are usually at a toddler's eye level, with safety caps. Unplug all kitchen or bathroom appliances that are not being used. And bind excess cord length from lamps and other electrical devices with a twist tie to prevent injury from chewing on cords.

To Prevent Drowning

Never leave a baby unattended in the bath. An infant can drown in only a few inches of water. Don't leave children unattended by a swimming pool, wading pool, or hot tub. Water wings, inflatable rings, and other floatation devices are not a substitute for constant adult supervision. Dump water out of wading pools when not in use.

To Prevent Cuts

Keep knives, forks, scissors, shaving razors, saws, and other sharp tools in a drawer with a safety latch or in a high cabinet. Keep glass drinking glasses or dishware far from a child's reach.

To Prevent Choking

Don't give a child under the age of four any hard foods that can block the windpipe. This includes cherries with pits, raw carrots, popcorn, and hard candy. Soft foods such as hot dogs, sausages, grapes, and caramels can also block a child's windpipe. Spoonfuls of peanut butter and chewing gum are also potential choking hazards. Never give balloons to a child younger than eight. Make sure you constantly check your children's toys for loose or broken parts.

To Prevent Animal Bites

Don't leave children less than a year old alone with the family dog, cat, or other pet. Until the age of four, they should be supervised when playing with a pet. Teach them never to tease an animal or to take food away from a dog.

Vaccines

Would you like to protect your child from some of the deadliest diseases in history? I'm sure you would. That's what vaccines do. But they also do a lot more than that. They protect your neighbors' kids and other children around the country at the same time; ultimately, if everyone follows suit, they'll rid the entire world of diseases that have been crippling and killing children for centuries. Vaccines are probably the most powerful health tools ever developed.

To understand why, you have to know a little bit about how your immune system works. Your immune system is an incredible defense mechanism. Whenever a virus invades your body, your immune system produces proteins called antibodies. These antibodies hunt down and destroy the viruses that make you sick. Since it takes your immune system a while to produce these antibodies, the first time a specific invader strikes, you'll get sick until the immune system has had a chance to catch up. But the antibodies that were produced from that first attack remain in your bloodstream forever; should the invader ever attack again, even years or decades later, these antibodies will come to your defense *before* you can get sick again. It's a great system. The only drawback is that you have to get sick once before you can develop that needed immunity from future attacks.

And that's where vaccines come into the picture. Vaccines work by giving your immune system just enough knowledge of a potential invader for your body to produce the antibodies it needs should the real virus ever attack—and the vaccine does so without getting you sick. Vaccines are made from a weakened or dead virus or the protein that encapsulates the virus. When the vaccine is injected into your system, your immune system reacts by producing antibodies, as if the actual disease were attacking it. These antibodies will give you immunity from any future attacks of the real disease.

Children today routinely receive twice as many vaccinations before kindergarten as they did a decade ago. Like any other medicine, vaccines will occasionally cause reactions, but these are usually mild, perhaps a slight fever or a soreness of the arm where the injection was given. More serious reactions are rare, but they do happen, and, as a consequence, some parents have developed a real fear of

Shoo, Flu!

The flu is caused by the influenza virus, which spreads from person to person through coughs and sneezes. Symptoms of the flu include fever, cough, sore throat, headache, chills, muscle aches, and fatigue. Anyone can get the flu, which for most people lasts a week or so. But some people are at high risk for complications from influenza, including convulsions, pneumonia, bronchitis, and the croup, which is a respiratory infection.

All children six to fifty-nine months of age are at high risk of complications because their immune systems are not fully developed. (People who have heart or lung disorders or chronic diseases such as diabetes, as well as people fifty years or older, are also at high risk and should get the flu shot.) Doctors recommend that children get their flu shots by October or earlier—before the flu season begins.

vaccines. One reason for these fears lies in the fact that some vaccines made since the 1930s contained thimerosal, a mercury-containing preservative that is used to kill live contaminants in vaccines. At high doses, mercury can cause irreversible nerve and brain damage, but definitely not in the doses found in vaccines. Nevertheless, today none of the vaccines used in the United States to protect preschool children against twelve infectious diseases contain thimerosal as a preservative, with the exception of some flu vaccines (see "Shoo, Flu!," page 34).

Protection from the Dirty Dozen

AGES OF SHOTS AND BOOSTERS *	DISEASE	VACCINE
Can vary according to blood type and other factors.		
12 months and ages 4 to 6 years	Measles, Mumps, Rubella (German measles)	MMR vaccine
2 months, 4 months, 6 months, 15 to 18 months, 4 to 6 years	Diphtheria, Tetanus (lockjaw), Pertussis (whooping cough)	DTaP vaccine
2 months, 4 months, 6 to 18 months, 4 to 6 years	Polio	Polio vaccine
2 months, 4 months, 6 months, 12 to 15 months	Haemophilus influenza type b (Hib disease)	Hib vaccine
Birth, 1 to 2 months, 6 to 18 months	Hepatitis B	Hepatitis B vaccine
12 to 24 months	Varicella (Chickenpox)	Varicella vaccine
12 months, 18 months	Hepatitis A	Hepatitis A vaccine
2 months, 4 months, 6 months, 12 to 15 months	Pneumococcal disease	Pneumococcal vaccine

Infectious Diseases

Common Cold—Too Common

The cold is the most common infectious disease in the United States, and it is the main reason for children to visit the doctor. We catch colds by breathing in rhinoviruses (*rhino* is the Greek word for nose) that are floating around in the air or by touching our mouth or nose after touching a surface contaminated with a rhinovirus. When these viruses penetrate the protective lining of the nose and throat, our immune system goes on the offense; the side effects of the battle are sore throat, headache, and runny or stuffy nose.

The best way to prevent a cold is to stay away from people who have one. That's not very easy to do, since a person coming down with a cold isn't aware of it to begin with and then doesn't try to advertise it afterward. To make matters worse, virus particles can travel up to twelve feet through the air when someone with a cold sneezes or coughs. We could reduce the incidence of colds if all cold sufferers simply cover their noses and mouths when they cough or sneeze, and wash their hands thoroughly and frequently, especially after blowing their noses.

THE COLD FACTS

Total number of colds each year in the United States:
   1,000,000,000
Number of colds per child per year: 6 to 10
Number of colds per adult per year: 2 to 4
Number of viruses known to cause the common cold: 200
Number of infected droplets in a single sneeze: 4,500
Speed at which droplets travel in miles per hour: 100

Cold Comforts

Although they won't necessarily cure you, here are a few measures you can take to make yourself feel better when you have a cold.

1. Chicken soup
There is no proof that this soup can cure a cold, though people have been using this remedy for hundreds of years. Chicken soup does contain an amino acid, however, that can help thin the mucus and perhaps in this way help control congestion.

2. Vitamin C, zinc, and echinacea
Researchers just aren't sure yet whether echinacea can help prevent a cold or whether vitamin C and zinc can help bring a cold to a quick conclusion. Studies have been inconclusive.

3. Feed a cold, starve a fever
Most doctors have rejected this as a myth. It doesn't help that sometimes the advice is given the other way around! On the other hand, Dutch scientists have found that eating a meal boosts the type of immune response that destroys the viruses responsible for colds, while fasting stimulates the response that tackles the bacterial infections responsible for most fevers. But it's only one study. So this one gets a maybe.

4. Over-the-counter decongestants and antihistamines.
There is little evidence that they actually work. In any case, these medicines must never be given to children under the age of two, as they can cause hallucinations, irritability, and irregular heartbeats in infants.

The symptoms of a cold usually appear two or three days after exposure to these nosy viruses and can last a week. There is little to do to treat a cold other than to get plenty of rest, drink lots of fluids, and let the cold run its course. To relieve muscle aches, headaches, and fever, you can give your child acetaminophen (Tylenol), but never give a child aspirin. (Giving aspirin to a child under twelve, or to a teen under nineteen who has a viral illness, can increase the risk of Reye's syndrome—which is a rare but serious illness that can be fatal.) But with colds being so darn common, lots of myths and folk remedies have arisen to fill medicine's inability to find a cure for the common cold (see "Cold Comforts," page 37). The evidence suggests, however, that they do little good, other than psychologically. But then thinking you're feeling better is nothing to sneeze at either.

Earaches

Ear infections rank number two after the cold as the most commonly diagnosed childhood illness in the United States. More than three out of four children will have one or more ear infections by their third birthday. Symptoms usually consist of severe ear pain and fever.

Most of the time, when the doctor diagnoses an ear infection, he or she is really talking about an infection of the middle ear. This part of the ear lies between the outer ear, where sound waves enter, and the inner ear, which translates vibrations into electric signals. The middle ear must be at the same pressure as the outer world to function properly, and this is taken care of by a small passage called the eustachian tube, which connects the middle ear to the back of the throat. Usually, this tube allows fluid to drain from the middle ear out into your throat, but if you get a virus or a bacteria that causes the tube to swell, the fluid from the middle ear can no longer drain normally. When the tube becomes blocked by congestion or by mucus due to a cold or an allergy, germs can breed in the trapped fluid and cause an ear infection.

Children develop ear infections more frequently between the ages of two and four for several reasons. Basically their eustachian tubes at that age are shorter, narrower, less stiff, and more horizontal than those of adults. This makes their tubes more prone to blockage and allows bacteria and viruses to find their way into the middle ear more easily than in adults. Also contributing to the problem is the fact that children have more trouble fighting off infections than adults do because children's immune systems are not fully developed until the age of seven. Then, to cap it off, almost literally, the adenoids, those glands in the back of the throat, are large in children and can block the opening of the eustachian tubes.

Most middle ear infections go away on their own within two or three days, or one or two weeks in the most severe cases. More and more doctors are recommending a wait-and-see approach to ear infections, rather than immediately prescribing antibiotics, as they have in the past. An overuse of antibiotics can lead to antibiotic-resistant bacteria, which could make the problem even more difficult to treat. Usually the pain and fever associated with ear infections can be controlled with acetaminophen or ibuprofen, and perhaps some pain-relieving eardrops, if the eardrum has not ruptured.

A few lifestyle choices can minimize the risk of children developing ear infections. Breast-feeding may prevent early episodes of ear infections, as does avoiding exposing children to tobacco smoke, which appears to increase the frequency and severity of ear infections. If your child is sick, do not take the child to day care; this will prevent the contamination of others. And remember to wash your hands and those of your child often.

It is important to pay attention to ear infections in young children because even though the infection doesn't cause a permanent hearing loss, it does produce a temporary hearing loss that may have serious consequences. Because young children learn how to speak by listening to sounds, imitating sounds, and hearing themselves make sounds, a temporary hearing loss could affect their speech development. If your child has more than three ear infections in six months, or four ear infections in a year, your doctor may suggest a low dose of antibiotics every day, especially during the winter season, while others may recommend a surgical procedure to place tubes in the ear to drain the middle ear.

It's Not Just for Girls

Pinkeye, or conjunctivitis, is the most common eye problem for kids. It usually involves a redness, itching, and swelling of the eyes, and is sometimes accompanied by a clear or colored discharge that collects in the corner of the eye. The same bacteria responsible for ear infections can cause conjunctivitis, but it can also be caused by a virus, in which case the antibiotic eyedrops the doctor will prescribe for this problem won't work. Kids will pick up pinkeye by playing around on the floor all day, then rubbing their eyes with dirty fingers. The best way to avoid pinkeye, which usually lasts less than a week, is by washing your child's hands with warm soapy water.

Even the Name is Contagious

Coxsackie. It's fun to say it, but it's not fun to get. The Coxsackie virus, which is named after the town in New York where is was first discovered, is a highly contagious stomach virus that is spread from person to person on unwashed hands and surfaces contaminated with feces. Oddly enough, half of all children who get Coxsackie have no symptoms. Others will develop headaches, muscle aches, and fevers up to 104°F. The hand, foot, and mouth version of the disease involves painful red blisters in the throat, on the tongue, on the insides of the cheeks, on the palms of the hands, and on the soles of the feet. The risk of infection is highest among infants and kids under the age of five. Outbreaks occur most frequently in the summer and fall in colder climates, and year-round in tropical climates. Since Coxsackie is a virus, antibiotics won't help. The best course of treatment includes acetaminophen to relieve the pain and fluids to prevent dehydration. If the fever lasts more than twenty-four hours and involves vomiting, difficulty breathing, or other serious symptoms, take your child to the doctor immediately.

Number Five?

Fifth disease makes its first appearance around the time kids start going to school, around age five, and they continue to be susceptible to it until about the age of fifteen. It's also called the slapped-cheek syndrome because children with this disease have rosy cheeks, as if they had been slapped in the face. The rash can last a couple of weeks and may spread to the trunk, arms, and legs, and be quite itchy. Fifth disease is actually just a viral illness caused by the parvovirus B19 and really can't be avoided. There is no treatment for it either, except supportive care and avoiding contact with other children, and most children recover from it quickly and without complications. It's name, by the way, stems from the fact that when diseases causing childhood rashes were enumerated, it was the fifth one listed. Duh, as the kids would say.

The Mother of All Sore Throats

Most sore throats are caused by viruses. A runny nose, cough, hoarseness, and runny eyes characterize these sore throats. More serious is strep throat, an infection caused by the A. *streptococci* bacteria that's usually present in the oral flora of the mouth. When it gets out of control, this bacteria produces fever, stomach pain, and red or swollen tonsils, as well as a severe sore throat.

To diagnose strep throat, the doctor will do a rapid strep test right in the office. This involves taking a sample of the fluids at the back of the child's throat with a swab. Five minutes later you'll know if the test is positive or negative. If it's negative, the doctor will probably send a sample to a lab for a culture to make sure that the negative was not a false reading. If it's positive, the doctor will probably prescribe a course of antibiotics for about ten days. Within twenty-four hours, the child's temperature will be back to normal and the child will be able to go back to school. Children must not go to school while infected with strep throat as the strep bacteria is highly contagious (it can even be spread by the family dog). A failure to treat a strep infection, or to complete the antibiotic treatment prescribed for it, can be serious; an untreated strep infection can lead to rheumatic fever, which can cause permanent damage to the heart, as well as scarlet fever or kidney disease.

When Hot Is Cool

Parents tend to worry excessively when their child's temperature rises above 98.6. They worry that a high fever will cause brain damage; they'll do a sponge bath or alcohol rubdown, or give their child an aspirin. But the reality is that a high fever won't cause brain damage; you don't need to do sponge baths or rubdowns; and whatever you do, you shouldn't give a child aspirin. Like the time of the Oldsmobile, the days of worrying about a fever are long past, but this idea is still deeply imbedded in the brains of most parents.

A high fever doesn't necessarily mean your child is very sick. A simple cold or virus can cause a high fever. On the other hand, a serious infection may not involve a fever at all, or it may even result in a low body temperature, which is especially likely to occur in young infants. The way your child is acting is far more important than the reading on the thermometer.

The fever itself does no harm. In fact, it shows that the body's immune system is working. Here's how: the body's temperature is regulated by the hypothalamus, a part of the brain that acts as the body's thermostat. The hypothalamus will raise the body's temperature in response to an infection or illness. Turning up the heat is the body's way of fighting viruses. The heat makes the body uncomfortable for the virus; unfortunately, it makes your child uncomfortable as well.

A fever should ring your alarm bells only if:

- An infant younger than three months has a temperature of 100.4°F or greater
- An older child has a fever greater than 104°F
- The fever lasts more than twenty-four hours in a child younger than two
- The fever lasts more than three days in an older child

Other reasons to call your doctor, regardless of how elevated the temperature, are if the child has difficulty breathing; is lethargic; cries inconsolably for hours; has persistent diarrhea; has blue lips, tongue, and nails; or has seizures.

Autism

Autism is not a disease or a mental illness. It is a developmental disability, though some people might find fault with that description and prefer to call it a neurological variation instead. In any case, it's a topic that's very important to me because I have an autistic child. I think that having an autistic child makes you a better parent overall because it doesn't allow you to take anything for granted. When you have a child who is autistic, you realize the importance of communication and how much you want to hear the words "I love you" from that child.

The mechanism of autism is still poorly understood, but clearly the incidence of autism has increased over the last decade. Where autism used to occur in fewer than five out of every ten thousand births, the number today is probably twice that, with some studies reporting that there may be twelve times that number of kids with some degree of autism per ten thousand births. Recently there has been a tremendous interest in finding the cause of this increase in autistic children. Some suspect a genetic influence, though no one has yet located an "autism gene." There is some evidence, in fact, that many factors may be involved in causing autism.

Other possible culprits include the mercury in childhood vaccinations. Mercury is present in small amounts in some vaccines to prevent bacterial contamination. While mercury is highly neurotoxic, the role it might play in autism is still being debated. Other suspects include lead poisoning in the environment, and pitocin, a drug given to pregnant women to induce labor. Still others point a finger to synthetic compounds like plastics and PCBs or food additives. The list of suspects goes on and on.

Autism may be apparent from birth. Infants may, for example, arch their back away from a caregiver to avoid physical contact. Others develop normally—sitting, crawling, and walking—until about the age of one and

Famous Autistics

Autism was once thought to be synonymous with mental retardation, or at least with low-functioning individuals. Nothing can be further from the truth. In fact, many individuals with a certain degree of autism have incredibly high IQs and are extraordinarily functional. Filmmaker Steven Spielberg is perhaps one of the most well-known individuals to be officially diagnosed with Asperger's syndrome, a mild version of autism. Other famous people suspected to have some degree of autism include Woody Allen, Bob Dylan, Bill Gates, and Al Gore. The list of people in history suspected of having some degree of autism include:

Albert Einstein	Emily Dickinson
Glenn Gould	Thomas Edison
Howard Hughes	Henry Ford
Thomas Jefferson	Thomas Jefferson
Wolfgang Amadeus Mozart	Carl Jung
Isaac Newton	Friedrich Nietzsche
J.R.R. Tolkien	Alfred Hitchcock
Alan Turing	Ayn Rand
Ludwig Wittgenstein	Socrates
Andy Warhol	Leonardo da Vinci
Jane Austen	Michelangelo
Ludwig van Beethoven	Charles Darwin
Alexander Graham Bell	Marie Curie

a half or so when their autistic symptoms begin to appear. These include repetitive, nongoal-directed behavior like rocking and hand flapping, as well as exhibiting poor eye contact, or throwing tantrums when routines are changed—this "insistence on sameness" is known as pervasive behavior. (Dustin Hoffman's character in the movie *Rainman* is a perfect example of pervasive behavior.)

Autism is four times more common in boys than in girls. No one knows why. Children also vary greatly in the nature and the severity of their disabilities. And because there are many forms of autism, there is no single way to describe someone who has autism. Some are antisocial; some are social. Some are aggressive toward others; some are aggressive toward themselves. While some have normal language skills, half of all autistic children have little or no language skills at all; they are unable to translate their thoughts into actions. Autistic children usually have problems with cognition; they are unable to realize that other people have their own unique point of view about the world. For example, an autistic child with cognition issues who is told to show a photograph of an animal to another child will not realize that the photograph has to be turned toward the other person for the person to see it.

The diagnosis of autism is usually applied to an individual who displays a number of characteristic autistic behaviors. This assessment is usually made by a pediatric neurologist, who will ensure that the child's behavior is not due to some other problem, like deafness, or to related but distinct diseases such as Fragile X syndrome, a genetic disorder that causes mental retardation, or Landau-Kleffner syndrome, a rare childhood neurological disorder characterized by the sudden loss of the ability to understand and use spoken language.

Once the diagnosis of autism is made, an intervention is planned. The intervention team usually consists of a pediatric neurologist, a physical therapist, an occupational therapist, and a behavioral therapist. The aim of this team is to begin to rebuild the communication pathways between the child's cognitive mind and behavioral expressions. This involves developing the child's auditory, visual, tactile, taste, vestibular, and olfactory senses. It may take years, but once these things are established, breakthroughs become possible. A child may then begin to speak and feel comfortable with his senses; he may cease to be hypersensitive; his attention may be more focused. Progressively the child becomes a more functional individual.

The challenge for parents of autistic children is to understand the importance of early intervention and the slow pace of success, and to appreciate that all these children are intelligent, highly motivated individuals who, with perseverance, make incredible sons and daughters. It's worth noting that autistic children who have siblings do much better than those who have no brothers and sisters.

Nutritional counseling needs to be a part of the evaluation of any autistic child; many autistic children are unable to break down certain proteins into amino acids. There are, for example, some reports of mild to dramatic improvements in the speech and behavior of autistic children after gluten and casein are removed from their diet. Gluten and glutenlike proteins are found in wheat and other grains, and are also found in starches, couscous, malt, vinegars, soy sauce, flavorings, and artificial colors. Casein is a protein found in milk and milk products and may also be present in such products as hot dogs. The use of vitamin B_6, magnesium, and other supplements may also have a beneficial effect.

Eventually, with lots of effort, the cognitive and sensory problems of an autistic child turn into a learning disability. The good schools that deal with these types of children have begun to integrate special classes with regular classes until—it might be in high school or it might be in college—the autistic individual is fully integrated into the regular system. Many colleges today—for instance, Boston University—have a special program for people who suffer from learning disabilities. The problem, however, is that many public-school systems cannot protect the rights of these kids by providing them the help they need. Unfortunately, in many parts of America working families do not have the resources—and neither do the states in which they live—to adequately teach these kids what they need to integrate into society.

There have always been autistic children. While severely autistic chil-

My son did not speak until the age of two. I was aware that he was atypical much earlier than that, but, of course, everybody said, No, he's fine, you're just being paranoid. My wife was convinced it was middle-child syndrome. He walked, he crawled, he cried, he drank, he was a beautiful baby. Then one day we had him tested, and, of course, he failed miserably. He was autistic.

I went crazy. I was depressed; I was angry at God. I said, How could you do this to me, I who deliver babies for a living? It took me a long time to accept it. But since I had the resources, I hired a team of professionals, and they did everything they could for my child. Five therapists, five hours a day, five days a week, nonstop. One would come in and another would leave, one would come in and another would leave. The tension in the house was horrible. My wife and I were at each other's throats.

Then one beautiful afternoon I was sitting in my office when one of the therapists called me and, almost in tears, said, "He spoke." Just like that. It took almost a year.

Now my son is eight. He still has pervasive development disorder (PDD), one of the many faces of autism, but he's a different kid. He'll say, "Daddy, I love you," or "Daddy, I'm very angry today." I desperately wanted to hear those words because I deeply believe that what defines us as human beings is our emotions, and that's far more important than anything else.

dren were once institutionalized, many of those who had milder forms of autism turned out to be our librarians, accountants, philosophers, and scientists. (See "Famous Autistics," page 44.) In other words, they were people who adapted themselves and were able to integrate into society. But because they never really felt comfortable around a lot of people, they didn't necessarily need highly developed communication skills.

A Whole Lot Going on Between the A and the D

Everybody's heard about it. Three little letters, or four, that mean trouble for your child. Attention deficit disorder (ADD), or attention deficit hyperactivity disorder (ADHD), typically gets noticed when the child goes to school for the first time. When kids are younger, say two or three years of age, they have had few social interactions with others, so many parents dismiss the problem, thinking, "They're just toddlers; they're just hyperactive." But when the child starts school, teachers may begin to notice that he or she cannot sit still and gets distracted very easily. There could be many reasons for ADHD, but it has nothing to do with cognitive functioning, or with whether the child is smart or not. It has to do with impulsive behavior, and it's very difficult to pinpoint because it's often misdiagnosed as simple misbehavior. But any child who is more impulsive and more hyperactive than other children of that age should be evaluated for ADHD.

Three to five percent of schoolchildren have ADHD. It usually first manifests by the age of seven, but it can last through childhood and into adulthood. Though not well understood, it tends to run in families. Usually about a quarter of parents of a child with ADHD have the disease themselves. When these types of behaviors are first noticed, parents should start a diary that keeps track of the child's behavior. This will be useful when the child is later evaluated by a team of certified specialists, usually an adolescent psychiatrist or a developmental pediatrician. Getting a proper evaluation is paramount because there are other things that a child could have in conjunction with ADHD, such as anxiety disorders, bipolar disorders, or even depression. An evaluation is also important because many of these children may have learning disabilities and will need the right tools to be able to keep up with their schoolwork.

If the diagnosis of ADHD is made, treatment may include behavioral therapy to control their aggression and modulate their social behavior, and cognitive therapy to help build up their self-esteem and reduce their negative thinking. Their school program may also need to be adjusted; they may need more time to complete a test, for instance, and they may need to be repositioned in the classroom so they are closer to the teacher.

Changes that require attention at home include modifying the way a parent deals with the ADHD child, by simplifying complex instructions. For example, hearing, "Pick up your room, wash your hands, and come down for dinner," can be confusing to an ADHD child. Parents may need to break down that interaction by giving the child one instruction at the time, letting him or her deal with it, and rewarding its accomplishment, before giving a second set of instructions.

Some children with ADHD will end up on medication. Medications can help improve their attention, focus, goal-directed behavior, and organizational skills. The prescribed medications vary widely, including antidepressants, but many individuals with ADHD are treated with stimulant medications, which seem to work by correcting a biochemical condition in the brain that interferes with attention and impulse control. The most commonly prescribed medication used to treat ADHD is Ritalin, though others include Adderall, Clonidine, Concerta, Strattera, Cylert, Wellbutrin, and Dexedrine. As with any medication, ADHD stimulant medications can produce such side effects in children as sleeping problems, stomachaches, headaches, drowsiness, irritability, nervousness, and, in rare cases, nervous tics, hallucinations, and bizarre behavior. That said, it should be noted that overall these medications seem to benefit about three-quarters of all children with ADHD.

As with most medications, those for ADHD should be taken only as long as it is helpful and necessary. With some children, the symptoms of ADHD will dissipate over time, and the medications will no longer be necessary. In others, the symptoms will persist into adolescence and young adulthood, and the medications will be required throughout.

The negative aspect of jumping into medication for ADHD is highlighted by the apparent rise of suicides in adolescents taking some of these medications. Although the jury's still out on whether there are direct links between suicidal tendencies in children taking ADHD medications, clearly many parent advocate groups are calling for stronger monitoring by the

ADD=ADHD?

"Dr. Manny, I'm confused. Our son is in his first year of elementary school, and he seems to have some attention problems. Some people are calling it ADD, and others are talking about it as ADHD. Are ADD and ADHD the same?"

The answer is yes and no. Attention deficit hyperactivity disorder, or ADHD, used to be known as attention deficit disorder, or ADD, and many people and professionals still use the term ADD. There really isn't a difference between the two terms as far as symptoms are concerned. Both can cause distractibility, forgetfulness, disorganization, difficulty following rapid conversations, and low self-esteem. The only real difference is that a person with ADD may be quiet and shy, whereas a person with ADHD will be hyperactive. So maybe the best way to think of it is that ADHD is just ADD with the added H.

FDA. So it is important for parents whose children are taking these medications to be aware of the fact that most of these drugs can have side effects. They should be alert to any atypical change in their child's behavior and always keep up a dialogue with the child, as well as with their primary care doctor.

Problems "Down There"

I don't need to tell you that boys and girls develop differently. Parents should be aware of their child's private parts from the very beginning and should make note of any changes they notice. Then as the child hits puberty, between eight and thirteen years of age, the parent should educate the child to be aware of his or her private parts so that he or she, too, can be aware of any changes or problems.

Young girls may develop vaginal problems. *Bacterial vaginitis* is very common in girls between the ages of two and four. It occurs when bacteria from the skin gets inside the vagina and causes irritation and inflammation. But it's nothing that proper hygiene can't prevent. It is important for mothers to teach their little girls how to wash themselves properly.

Vaginal itching is extremely common in young girls. A child with *vulvovaginitis,* as it is formally known, will scratch her vaginal area or complain of burning or pain when she urinates. Before puberty, the skin around the vaginal area can be very sensitive and become red and inflamed by a number of common irritants. One of the most common is soap or shampoo. A lot of young children take bubble baths, and parents tend to forget to rinse them properly after they sit and play in the soap suds. Another common reason is poor toilet hygiene. When toilet training young girls, parents must also teach them to wipe after urination, which sometimes they forget to do in all the excitement over their success in having them sit on the potty. On the other hand, excessive wiping after urination can also cause irritation and itching.

In rare cases, vaginal itching can be associated with pinworms, which look like small pieces of thread and are about a quarter of an inch long. Usually pinworms cause itching around the anal area, but they can also manifest in the lower vagina. Pinworms tend to cause symptoms at night when they migrate out of the anal area. If recognized, pinworms are diagnosed very easily with fecal cultures and are easily treatable. See your doctor for this.

As young girls approach the age of eight or nine, vaginal itches may be caused by *vaginal yeast infections.* Yeast is a natural flora of the vaginal mucosa, but when it overgrows, it can lead to an inflammation, causing burning, redness, and irritation, and it may produce a thick white discharge. There are many reasons for the overgrowth of vaginal yeast. The routine use of antibiotics, which may occur in children with frequent ear infections and throat infections, can lead to the overgrowth of yeast in the vaginal area. Poor hygiene, again, can be another reason. Even a small piece of toilet paper left in the small vaginal orifice can cause an infection and vaginal itching. A diaper rash in infants and toddlers may appear not only in the buttocks and anal area, but also in the vaginal area, and that could also be attributed to an overgrowth of yeast. Most of these problems are easily treated either by a primary care physician or by a pediatrician.

Urinary tract infections are, of course, a recurring issue for women during their entire lives. The reason why women get more urinary tract infections is because the tube that connects their bladder to the outside, called the *urethra,* is very short. This means that bacteria can make their way into the bladder fairly easily. Males don't have this problem as often because the penis provides them with a longer urethra.

Girls can also have something called *bladder reflux,* in which the urine flow from the bladder backs up into the tubes called *ureters,* instead of flowing normally down from the kidneys, through the ureters, to the bladder. This problem is commonly diagnosed in children who have had a urinary tract infection. The infection can cause a blockage in the urinary system, which then leads to a swelling of the ureter.

Males, on the other hand, may experience problems with their testicles. One is *varicoceles,* which is essentially a varicose vein within the testicle. It's caused by a damaged valve in the vein, draining blood from the testicle. There is nothing that can be done to prevent it, and there is no treatment, although if the boy is uncomfortable, he may need to wear supportive underwear.

Then there is *testicular torsion,* which may occur beginning at the age of eight or nine. The problem causes an acute severe pain of the testicles, or sometimes just a dull pain. Testicular torsion is a twisting of the spermatic cord that holds each testicle suspended within the scrotum. When the cord becomes twisted, it can cut off the blood supply to a testicle. If it is not treated quickly (within hours), the boy could lose a testicle; an operation may be needed to untwist the cord. There is no known cause for testicular torsion, but it can sometimes result from physical activity.

A third problem are *inguinal hernias,* which are basically weaknesses or tears in the wall of the groin. Though not confined to boys, boys will experience inguinal hernias about ten times more frequently than girls. Symptoms include pain, nausea, blocked bowels, and a bulge in the groin area, which can extend to the scrotum in boys, that remains even when lying down. Surgery is usually necessary to repair the hernia.

Both girls and boys are subject to *precocious puberty.* This occurs when signs of puberty appear prematurely—with breast development and the onset of menstruation in girls before age seven or eight, or with the enlargement of the testis and penis and facial and pubic hair growth in boys before the age of nine. When it occurs in girls, there is usually no underlying medical problem, though there may be one in boys, in whom the condition is less common but may be hereditary. Hormones in food, especially hormone-grown poultry and beef, may cause early development in girls, according to some reports. Precocious puberty can be physically and emotionally difficult for children. It's important that parents provide a supportive environment for the sexually precocious child, explaining that these changes are normal for older kids and teens, but that his or her body has started developing a little too early.

It's All in Your Hands—Parenting

Having kids is a big responsibility. Parenting is not a passive activity. What you do in that first decade of your child's life, and particularly in those first five or six years, has a big impact on how he or she will do when encountering the speed bumps of the second decade, such as depression, obesity, and anorexia. If you don't play with your children, if you don't talk to them, if you treat them badly, you will be adversely affecting the rest of their lives. And if as parents you are not reasonably good models of behavior, your children will imitate you and turn out to be troublesome kids as well.

Parents must teach their children good behavior so that they can mature into healthy intelligent young people. The best way to teach them good behavior is not by preaching to them but by setting an example. That's what kids know how to do best—they imitate, and the people they are most likely to imitate in the first decade of their lives are their parents. When bad behavior occurs, correct it right away. But it's also very important to notice and encourage their good behavior. If children don't get your attention for their good behavior, they know they can count on getting it for their bad behavior.

Become involved in your child's daily activities. Play with your children. It's a great opportunity to identify their needs and abilities and to teach them positive behavior as well as improve their social skills. When playing, let them take the lead to build up their self-esteem. Make a game out of following instructions; this will make it easier the next time you tell them to stop doing something they shouldn't be doing. But most important of all, remember to keep it real. Be reasonable when setting expectations for toddlers and preschoolers. They're only just beginning to learn.

Test Checklist for this Decade

	APGAR test
	Vaccines
	Vision and hearing tests
	Physical exam (BMI, etc., yearly)
	Yearly dental visit (once adult molars appear)

Life Is Beautiful

2

(The Second Decade: Ages 10 to 19)

You are now your own person.
These are exciting times.
You become aware of your body, of its incredible
power. You feel invincible. Life is beautiful.
But you may tend to overdo things at bit,
and at times life can feel a little too intense.
Don't let it spiral out of control.
You are now responsible for your own health.
And you wouldn't want it any other way.

I think today's American teenagers are wonderful. Why do I say that? Because when I compare my teenage self with this generation, I find that teens today are more mature, have a stronger sense of social justice, and are much better informed on current events. One thing I've noticed is that if you empower a teen with good morals and a loving and responsible home environment, you are going to end up with a very special individual.

That's why I found a recent study from the U.S. National Institute of Child Health and Human Development (NICHD) so disheartening. The study concluded that by the time American teenagers reach early adulthood, most have already adopted at least one unhealthy behavior: smoking, overeating, or abusing alcohol. The saddest part about it is that it doesn't have to be that way. With proper parental care, all these behaviors can be avoided. Some problems may strike in this decade regardless of a teen's behavior; however, they are especially likely to occur if the child wasn't properly prepared for them in the first decade of life. One of these problems has to do with seasonal allergies.

Ah-Choo!

Forty percent of U.S. children have seasonal allergies. When a parent has allergies, his or her child will probably have them, too. Most allergies tend to appear in childhood. So if you have seasonal allergies as an adult, you probably started getting them as a kid. As children, boys get more allergies than girls, but as they get older women usually catch up to the men. Even though we say that allergies are seasonal, they can occur year-round. In

Sweet Advice

Research has shown that a few spoonfuls of honey might provide some relief from the miserable symptoms of seasonal allergies. How so? It's basically the immune system's take on an old saw: familiarity breeds contempt. It turns out that local honey is rich in the same pesky pollens that make people sneeze, because honey-generating bees pick up pollen as they buzz around from plant to plant. So the idea is that by ingesting the local pollen in honey, we can potentially stop our immune system from reacting so severely when we inhale pollen in the springtime air. What people who try this remedy tend to forget, however, is that the honey must be local, meaning it has to come from the place where you live. In other words, if you live in Connecticut and you get allergies in Connecticut, buying honey from Oregon won't solve your problem. Check with your pediatrician before giving honey to very young children, however.

the spring you can get allergies to grass and pollen, and in the fall you can get allergies to ragweed and molds and spores of different kinds.

Allergies occur when pollen, mold, or dust kick your immune system into high gear, triggering a release of histamines, those chemicals that are mostly responsible for the sneezing, the runny nose, the itchy throat, and the watery eyes. If teenagers weren't properly exposed to their environment as children, their immune system won't be able to recognize as harmless the pollen, dust, and mold spores around them every day. (See "Loading the Virus Protection Program," page 29.)

Prevention is the best treatment for seasonal allergies. Have you heard of spring cleaning? They don't call it that for nothing. If people in your household have allergies, it is important to do a thorough cleaning of the house, especially in the spring, by removing all the dust that has collected in your house over the winter. It's a good time to shampoo your rugs, vacuum all the nooks and crannies, and remove the mold from all kitchen, bathroom, and garage surfaces. If you have allergies in the spring and summer, take a few precautionary steps to avoid bringing allergens back into the house. When you come in from the outdoors, don't bring the clothes you've worn outdoors into the bedroom; change in another part of the house and take a shower, if you can. Avoid being outdoors from the late morning to early afternoon, as those are the peak hours for pollen production. Keep your windows closed if you're really allergic.

Ask Dr. Manny

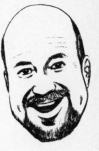

IS IT A COLD OR AN ALLERGY?

"Dr. Manny, how do you doctors do it? How do I know if my child has a cold or an allergy? It seems to me they both give you a runny nose and make you sneeze. Can you let us in on the secret?"

You're right, the symptoms of an allergy and the common cold are much the same. Both can produce a runny nose, sneezing, watery eyes, an itchy throat, and a headache. But there are several fundamental differences between the two. In colds the discharge from a runny nose will start out clear before turning green or yellow after three to five days. Allergies tend to produce a clear discharge from a runny nose throughout the allergic period. With a cold, you usually get better within ten to fourteen days, while allergy symptoms can continue unchecked for months. Children with colds might have fevers and muscle aches, but you typically won't see this with allergies. When one member of a family has a cold, other members of the family usually catch it, too. That's usually not the case with allergies, unless the whole family suffers from them. Children with allergies have dark circles under their eyes called shiners, a symptom that's not typically seen in colds. Of course, a doctor can tell if your child has a cold by looking at the nasal mucosa, the tissue that lines the nasal cavity. With an allergy, the nasal mucosa is usually pale and swollen; in a cold it's usually red and inflamed.

Allergies are usually treated with antihistamines, which reduce the symptoms but don't cure or prevent allergies. Commonly used antihistamines include Claritin, Zyrtec, and Allegra. Sometimes nonsteroidal medications like Rhinocort or Flonase are used to combat allergies. If your child has serious seasonal allergies, have him or her tested to identify exactly what makes the child allergic.

Asthma

Asthma is not only the most common chronic childhood disease, it is also the most misunderstood. Five million kids under the age of eighteen have asthma. More than three hundred people die of asthma each year. Asthma is on the rise in the United States, though it's not clear why. It's more common in young boys than in girls until the numbers even out in the teenage years. And it's more prevalent among blacks and city dwellers than among whites and those who live in suburban and rural areas.

Asthma is a chronic disease caused by a temporary inflammation of the smallest of our breathing tubes, called *bronchi* and *bronchioles,* that branch out from our windpipe. This inflammation causes a narrowing of the airways, which eventually become blocked through the buildup of mucus. The classic symptoms of asthma are easily recognizable: shortness of breath, wheezing, and a tight feeling in the chest. When these symptoms persist or become more severe, emergency treatment may be necessary to restore normal breathing.

Though the precise mechanism that causes asthma is not clearly understood, there clearly are trigger mechanisms that set it off, just as there are in seasonal allergies. Dust mites, mold, pollen, animal dander, and cockroach debris can all trigger asthma. Other factors—such as cold air, exercise, and stress—can also promote an asthmatic attack. Kids with food allergies are more prone to develop asthma, and viral infections such as respiratory syncytial virus and parainfluenza virus can also cause the inflammations that trigger asthma. Asthma also tends to be hereditary.

The list of apparent asthma triggers goes on and on. Tobacco smoke is a big problem. A parent who smokes around a child puts that child at risk for developing asthma. In fact, passive smoking is thought to cause as many as twenty-six thousand new cases of asthma each year. Still other triggers for asthma involve paint fumes, pollution, and perfume sprays.

Even humidity and sudden weather changes can produce an asthmatic attack.

If removing the environmental triggers for asthma proves either impossible or ineffective, two types of medication are used to relieve its symptoms. Anti-inflammatory drugs, like steroids, are used to control the inflammation of the airways, the swelling and mucous production, in other words. These drugs make the airways less sensitive and likely to react to the various asthma triggers. The other kind of asthma medication is the bronchodilator. These are usually inhalers that bring quick relief of the symptoms, often within minutes, by relaxing the muscles around the airways and making breathing easier. Such asthma treatments usually follow a stepwise approach. That means that you start with the lowest dose of effective medication and subsequently step up the dose and frequency as the asthma get worse.

The most important thing for parents to know is that there is no reason to be afraid of asthma. Become involved and educated about asthma because the best possible way to control asthmatic attacks is by learning to recognize the symptoms, getting effective treatment early on, and creating an environment for your child with fewer trigger mechanisms in order to reduce the frequency of attacks. Some people are able to outgrow their asthma, especially in mild cases or in those cases that are induced by exercise. But for most asthma sufferers, it's a disease that sticks around for life.

Acne

Acne is the scourge of youth. If you had it, you know exactly how miserable it felt to have all those little red and white bumps and scars on your face, and how helpless you were to prevent them. People of all races get acne, boys as well as girls. It usually starts at the age of eleven, though outbreaks can appear up until the age of thirty, and some people suffer from it into their forties and fifties.

Busting Acne Myths

Chocolate causes acne—FALSE
Greasy foods cause acne—FALSE
Dirty skin causes acne—FALSE

Those should actually be "False, but . . ." statements. Doctors will say that there is little evidence (meaning there is some evidence) that foods have much of an effect on the development and course of acne in most people (meaning that it can in some people). And while dirty skin will not cause acne, it can promote bacteria and cause infections in acne lesions that may have been picked at by the acne sufferer.

Acne is not a health threat, but it can cause significant emotional distress for adolescents—as well as for their parents. A field guide of acne lesions would include everything from *pustules,* or simple pimples, to *papules,* or small pink bumps on the skin that are tender to the touch, to very large *nodules,* which are painful solid lesions locked deep in the skin, to *cysts,* those deep, painful, pus-filled lesions that can cause scarring.

Knowing what acne is doesn't make it any better, but I'll tell you anyway. What we know about acne is that it results from the actions of hormones on the skin's oil glands. An excess of oily secretions clogs up the skin's pores and produces bacterial outbreaks that we call zits or pimples. Acne can affect any part of the human body, including the back, chest, and shoulders, though we mostly tend to think of acne as a facial problem because that's where the problem is most visible.

Other than the role of hormones, and in particular the male hormone, androgen, the exact cause of acne is not known. During puberty there is an increase in the androgen hormone in both boys and in girls,* causing the oil glands to enlarge and produce more oil. Genetics are thought to play a factor in acne, so if one or both parents had acne, the child probably will, too. Sometimes the early use of cosmetics can lead to the premature clogging of skin follicles, worsening an acne condition. The changes in hormone levels in adolescent girls two to seven days before a menstrual

* A male hormone in girls? Yes, androgen is the male sex hormone that controls the development of male characteristics, but it also is the precursor of estrogen, which is the female sex hormone.

period can also trigger an outbreak. So can backpacks and sports equipment, like tight helmets. Hard scrubbing of the skin, especially young skin, can lead to acne, too. So can stress, which is, again, a very common problem in the teen years.

If not treated adequately, acne can lead to scarring of the skin. So the goal of treatment is to heal the existing lesions, stop new lesions from forming, and minimize the psychological stress and embarrassment acne causes. All the medications available for acne basically attempt to decrease the oil production, the inflammation, and any secondary infection caused when bacteria is trapped under the skin. These medicines range from over-the-counter to prescription and involve both pills and creams. Commonly used over-the-counter products for mild inflammatory acne include benzoyl peroxide and salicylic acid. For more moderate to severe inflammation there are topical antibiotics and vitamin A-derived medicines, like Retin-A. For severe acne infection doctors will prescribe oral medicines, commonly Accutane, which is extremely dangerous for women who are pregnant and should be taken *only* under strict medical supervision.

What instructions should we give our kids about taking care of their skin properly? One is to gently clean their skin, especially the face, once in the morning and once in the evening, and also after strenuous exercise. Avoid using strong soaps or rough scrubs, especially on young skin. For boys, it's a good idea not to introduce shaving before it's necessary, though young boys are always eager to experiment with their fathers' shavers. For girls, hold

Risks of Accutane

Offered as treatment for serious cases of acne, Accutane is a synthetic form of vitamin A, and many of the side effects of Accutane resemble the side effects from an overdose of vitamin A.

Among the serious and potentially life-threatening risks associated with Accutane are birth defects, kidney failure, heart problems, and death. According to the FDA, Accutane may also cause violent behaviors, depression, psychosis, and, rarely, suicide.

Accutane is regarded as a "last choice" treatment for patients who have not responded to conventional acne therapies such as antibiotics. In early 2006, the FDA initiated the iPledge program, which requires registration of drug providers, health-care providers, and patients who want to use Accutane. Patients who are prescribed Accutane now have to agree to be monitored.

off on the use of cosmetics; once they do start using them, choose them carefully: always make sure they are oil-free. Teenagers should avoid sunburns, which can damage the skin and cause even small lesions to grow and become a major problem. Don't wait to get treatment for acne. It's a tremendously difficult condition, and it can put unnecessary strain on your teenager's life. Many treatment options exist, and often results are quick to come by. Be nice to your skin—remember, it's got you covered.

Our Supersized Kids (Obesity)

Obesity is perhaps the most serious health threat to children and adolescents from ages ten to sixteen. It is now, in fact, a worldwide epidemic. The number of overweight and obese children and adolescents has tripled in the past twenty-five years. In the United States more than 30 percent of children and adolescents are now overweight, and more than 15 percent are obese. Studies show that nearly three out of four overweight and obese kids will be overweight and obese as adults, which shows just how difficult it is to overcome obesity. These children will be sicker as they get older, more likely to suffer from heart disease, stroke, and diabetes than children of normal weight. How severe is this problem? Health experts believe that today's kids will be the first generation with a lower life expectancy than their parents. That is simply frightening.

How this happened is no secret.

There are four main reasons why obesity is a major health issue today: an increasing dependence on prepared foods, a tendency to eat too much, insufficient exercise, and gestational diabetes.

Food Preparation

The way we prepare most of our food has changed dramatically over the past couple of decades. We have gone from home-cooked meals using many fresh-from-the-garden ingredients to mass-market meals of store-bought processed foods. The processed-food industry has exploded in the past decade in particular. Statistics show that nearly a third of family meals nationwide are now prepared outside the home. That's a huge number. It's a reality of modern life that parents sometimes just don't have time to cook. So the marketplace has made it easier and easier for consumers to find products to eat.

What is the difference between a processed meal and a meal prepared at home? It's a matter of nutritional values. There is a fundamental difference between freshly prepared foods and processed foods: fresh foods retain their nutritional values while processed foods usually contain preservatives and trans-fatty acids to increase the product's shelf life, high sodium content to make it tasty, and other ingredients that may make it look good but that might not be particularly good for you.* Many of these foods are high in calories and fat. So many people who live on fast food, microwavable meals, and other prepackaged meals are actually malnourished. Nothing better illustrates this than the fact that some obese children are found to have rickets, a nutritional deficiency traditionally associated with starvation.

The consumption of processed foods has had a tremendous impact on the nutritional value of the food we eat and feed our children. The Ameri-

Corn-Fed Reality

In the 1980s, high fructose corn syrup replaced sugar in sodas because corn is cheaper than sugar. Since then, corn stripped to its building blocks and reassembled into sweeteners, stabilizers, and preservatives is now present in just about everything we eat—and use. That means that corn is not only in frozen yogurt, cake mixes, soups, ketchup, nondairy creamers, and, of course, candies, but it's also in toothpaste, disposable diapers, and more. Much more. How much more? Would you believe that more than a quarter of the forty-five thousand items in an average American supermarket contain corn? There is nothing wrong with corn itself, of course. It's when we extract the sugars from corn, which are high in calories, and consume food products made of this high fructose corn syrup that corn contributes to the obesity epidemic.

---

* Trans fats are exceptionally bad for you because your body treats them as if they were saturated fats, which raise your bad cholesterol and can lead to clogged arteries and heart disease.

Why Is Junk Food Junk?

Junk food is junk because it's food with a limited nutritional value. The calories it provides are, in fact, empty calories, but don't think for a minute that means calorie-free; it's just the opposite. If the first two ingredients in a food product are fat and sugar—you can be sure it's genuine junk food. Read that ingredients list carefully. Sugars can hide under a variety of names, including sucrose, dextrose, honey, fructose, maltose, high fructose corn syrup, lactose, glucose, molasses, corn syrup, corn sweetener, and brown sugar. The fats to look out for are saturated fats and hydrogenated oils, which are among the worst possible things you can put into your body. Junk foods also often have a high salt content. What's so bad about salt? If our salt levels are too high, our bodies retain too much fluid, which can lead to high blood pressure, and which in turn increases the risk of coronary heart disease and stroke. However, none of these substances, when used in moderation, can make you sick; it is only when we take them excessively that problems arise.

can diet, especially in the last twenty to thirty years, has become rich in refined carbohydrates—the pastas, flours, and sweets we just can't seem to get enough of. This diet means that the number of calories we consume daily has increased dramatically over the past few decades. We consume 25 percent more calories today, that is, an extra 530 calories per person per day, than we did thirty years ago. That's one reason why we have this obesity crisis.

Overeating

It's not just what we eat, but how much we eat. We, as a society, value quantity. American industry has made us desire the biggest cars, the widest television screens, and the largest homes. We are a society where size matters, and this appetite for the biggest, the largest, has been successfully applied to what we eat and drink as well. Portion sizes have steadily increased for both ready-to-eat and restaurant meals over the years. We value restaurants that serve big portions. Fifty years ago, soft drinks came in six-and-a-half-ounce bottles. Today soft drinks come in twenty- and thirty-two-ounce bottles. We don't buy a mere cheeseburger anymore, we buy at least a double cheeseburger. In many fast-food restaurants, a single "supersized" or "extra-value" meal provides more than an entire day's worth of calories.

What we have to come to grips with is the fact that less is better. We need to consume fewer calories than we do today in order to regain our health as a nation. That's going to be a hard sell, because after getting used to bigger is better, the idea that less is better is going to be difficult to swallow. But the fact is, there is a limit to how much our bodies can consume. You can't put fifty gallons of gasoline in your car when your tank holds only twenty gallons, because it's going to spill over the outside of the car and ruin the paint. Well, right now our bodies are being ruined because we stuff more calories into them than we can burn.

What Exercise?

Food preparation and extra calories are two parts of the obesity equation. A lack of exercise is the third factor in this growing epidemic. By "exercise" I'm not talking about going to the gym to work out. I'm talking about the kind of routine daily exercise we used to do that we no longer do. We have gone from walking to work and walking to school, for example, to taking a car to work or taking a bus to school, from performing physical tasks at work to doing mostly information-processing tasks that involve little or virtually no physical movement. As a society, we have minimized our physical activities dramatically, and that has had a tremendous impact on our ability to burn calories. So not only are we now consuming more calories—and often the wrong kinds of calories—but we're also doing less physical activity. And that, of course, is creating more overweight people.

Three social phenomena have converged recently to make this problem even worse for our children. Number one is that schools, for the most part, don't place much emphasis on physical education. Less than a third of students in grades nine through twelve engage in moderate physical activity at least thirty minutes a day, five or more days a week. Some states don't even require physical education at all in public schools, and it's not a priority in most states. Only one state, Illinois, requires all students to take a physical education class every day. That's how it should be in every state. Physical education should be part of every school curriculum, even from an early age.

The second social phenomenon responsible for the growing number of obese children is the increase in sedentary behavior caused by television, video games, and computers. Yes, television stimulates our visual sense, video games increase our dexterity, and computers make a world of facts and figures available to us at the touch of a mouse, but for all the benefits of these technologies, they have also allowed children to occupy more of their time with yet another sedentary activity. More than a quarter of all children in grades nine through twelve watch more than four hours of TV a day, and two-thirds of them watch more than two hours of TV a day. Could a reduction in TV-watching time have an effect on a child's weight? Absolutely. Some studies show that a decrease in television watching and playing with video games can lead to a decrease in a child's body mass index (BMI). (See "The Best Measure of Weight [BMI]," page 69.)

The third social phenomenon that makes the situation even worse is the fact that during all those hours of watching TV we are bombarded by advertisements for foods that, nutritionally speaking, leave a lot to be desired. The more TV we watch, the greater the chances are that our food choices will be determined by TV advertising. And what foods do we see advertised on television? Broccoli? Brown rice? Bananas? Definitely not. Most TV advertising is food with questionable nutritional value. Studies show that most ads shown during children-viewing hours, in fact, are for sugary breakfast cereals, candy snacks, and fast food. One study in Boston showed that children who watched more television consumed an extra 167 calories per additional hour of television watched. So instead of watching what we eat, we are eating what we watch.

A recent trend in TV advertising has made an already awful situation absolutely disastrous. It's called *cobranding,* or advertising that links the icons of popular culture with products such as sneakers or fast food. Buying sneakers can't hurt you (though it can hurt your pocketbook), but buying food that's bad for you is an entirely different matter. I find it totally irresponsible that the food industry is now putting cartoon characters on packaging for ice creams and cereals that are essentially pure sugar

The Big Camp

Children's obesity camps and spas are opening all over America. Unfortunately, these places are very crowded. These camps constitute a huge business now because there's such a high demand for them. The good ones are operated by pediatricians who will give children a thorough evaluation of their physical needs. In other words, they calculate the children's BMI (see "The Best Measure of Weight [BMI]," page 69) and review their medical history. The kids then participate in physical activities under the guidance of an instructor. All the machines are designed with children in mind: the bicycles are for children, the treadmills are for children, the weight machines are for children, and a lot of them will be linked to video games. But in order for them to play the video games, they have to peddle the bicycle or whatever machine they are on. It works because kids then want to go to the gym, and they begin to understand the importance of exercise. These places also teach kids the importance of nutrition—that eating is not just a matter of consuming foods that taste good; rather, it's a way of making their bodies healthier. They learn what calories are, what fats and proteins are, what carbohydrates are, and what foods provide good nutritive value.

and have no nutritional value, and then pricing these products in such a way that even the poorest of parents can afford them. We have to demand that the food industry respect our efforts to reverse obesity and that it stop creating venues of cobranding that target kids with advertisements for junk foods. This *must* stop right now. If industry wants to paste cartoon characters on bananas and broccoli stems, that's okay with me, but they must not do so on foods that will exacerbate our current obesity crisis.

Fat Lifestyles

The fourth factor responsible for the obesity epidemic in this country is the increase in gestational diabetes. Diabetic mothers deliver large babies. So right from the get-go most of the children coming into the world today are of a significant weight. And things usually don't get any better after that. A lot of doctors are saying, "fat parents, fat household, fat kid," and they are right. Studies have shown that 70 percent of obese children will also be obese as adults. The transition is linear. So nearly three quarters of the time, what you are today as a child is what you're going to be as an adult.

A fat family tends to stays fat. The most important individual when it comes to a child's health is not the doctor, the teacher, or the minister. It's the parent(s). Studies have shown that if you try to change the eating habits of a child when you yourself have poor eating habits, it just doesn't work. You cannot force a child to eat a balanced diet—to enjoy vegetables, or think of food not as a reward or as a product that tastes good, but rather as a nutrient and fuel for the body—if you don't think and act that way as a parent. You cannot force a kid to exercise when you yourself don't exercise. And don't think for a minute that an overweight child will just outgrow his or her weight; it won't happen by itself.

The Best Measure of Weight (BMI)

Being overweight is not just a matter of weight. That's an old-fashioned notion. The best measure that physicians and researchers currently use takes into account both height and weight in a formula that results in what is called the body mass index, or BMI for short. The BMI number is really the percent of fat in your body. The formula for calculating BMI is simple:

$$BMI = \frac{\text{weight in pounds}}{\text{height in inches x height in inches}} \times 703$$

But since a child's body fat changes as he or she grows over the years, and boys and girls differ in their body fat as they mature, the BMI for children is both age and gender specific. After calculating your child's BMI, find the number on the boy or girl's BMI-for-age charts, which apply to ages two to twenty.

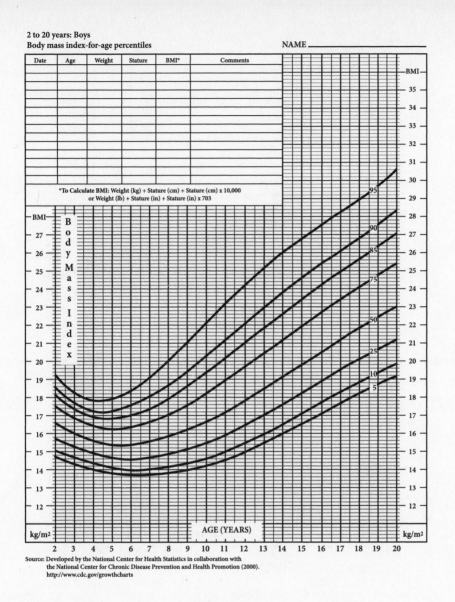

2 to 20 years: Boys
Body mass index-for-age percentiles

NAME _____

Date	Age	Weight	Stature	BMI*	Comments

*To Calculate BMI: Weight (kg) + Stature (cm) + Stature (cm) x 10,000
or Weight (lb) + Stature (in) + Stature (in) x 703

Body Mass Index

AGE (YEARS)

kg/m²

Source: Developed by the National Center for Health Statistics in collaboration with
the National Center for Chronic Disease Prevention and Health Promotion (2000).
http://www.cdc.gov/growthcharts

To eradicate childhood obesity, parents will have to lead by example. They have to play an active role by losing weight and being examples of good health habits themselves. By doing so, parents can change the whole dynamic of the household. Children and parents should go grocery shop-

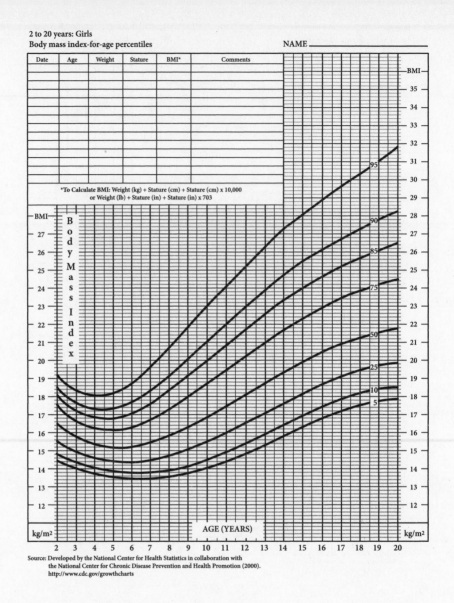

2 to 20 years: Girls
Body mass index-for-age percentiles

NAME _____

Date	Age	Weight	Stature	BMI*	Comments

*To Calculate BMI: Weight (kg) ÷ Stature (cm) ÷ Stature (cm) x 10,000
or Weight (lb) ÷ Stature (in) ÷ Stature (in) x 703

AGE (YEARS)

Source: Developed by the National Center for Health Statistics in collaboration with
the National Center for Chronic Disease Prevention and Health Promotion (2000).
http://www.cdc.gov/growthcharts

UNDERWEIGHT: If the BMI is less than the 5th percentile

NORMAL: If the BMI is between the 5th and the 85th percentile

AT RISK OF BEING OVERWEIGHT: If the BMI is between the 85th and 95th percentile

OVERWEIGHT: If the BMI is greater than the 95th percentile

ping together to learn how to pick the right foods—including fruits and vegetables—for the family. Children and parents should cook together so that they learn how to prepare food in a healthy way. Children and parents should exercise together, creating windows in their week during which exercise, or some form of physical activity, is incorporated into their regular routines. Whether you take walks in the afternoon together or you spend quality time in the backyard throwing a baseball around, it's important to make exercise a habit. If you don't do all of this together, in the end obesity will win out. The parent must assume the leadership position and say: No, we're not going to be fat; we're going to eat healthy, and we're *all* going to do it. This is the only way that we can make a difference.

The Fit States and Couch Potato States

Child Magazine recently ranked the best and worst states based on twenty health factors related to exercise and nutrition. These included requirements for physical education, number of parks and playgrounds, number of fast-food restaurants, and school-nutrition policies. The best state was Connecticut. The worst was Alaska.

Top Ten States for Raising Healthy Children

1. Connecticut
2. New York
3. Vermont
4. Massachusetts
5. Missouri
6. Maine
7. West Virginia
8. Wisconsin
9. Arkansas
10. Illinois

Ten Worst States for Raising Healthy Children

41. Iowa
42. Wyoming
43. Idaho
44. Alabama
45. South Dakota
46. Kansas
47. Mississippi
48. Nevada
49. Nebraska
50. Alaska

Eat Less, Move More

Poor weight control has serious consequences. It can lead to an increase in heart disease, high blood pressure, risk of cancer, breathing problems, arthritis, reproductive complications, gallbladder disease, and, of course, Type 2 diabetes. There are two types of diabetes, Type 1 and Type 2. In Type 1 the pancreas doesn't produce enough insulin to break down sugars; it's a genetic problem (see "Diabetes—Type 1," page 75.) But the vast majority of diabetics, that is, more than 90 percent, are Type 2, which is brought on by being overweight; it's an abnormality in glucose metabolism (see "Diabetes Again," page 212). Until recently, Type 2 diabetes was a disease seen only in older, overweight adults. Fifteen years ago we had never ever seen a child with Type 2 diabetes. Now, 25 percent of the cases of Type 2 diabetes occur in children. Diabetes is a serious disease. It is the leading cause of blindness, the leading cause of kidney failure, and the leading cause of nontraumatic amputation in the United States.

We can tackle childhood obesity. All we have to do is consume fewer calories, make those calories healthy ones, and then burn the calories we do consume through exercise. It's really that simple. Do that, and we can change a whole generation.

Dental Health

The decade with the most dental problems? One guess: the teens. That's not a big surprise, of course. The high sugar consumption during the teenage years results in significant tooth decay, and that means more cavities, more gingivitis (gum disease), and more root canals than in any other age group until the senior years.

The problem is made worse by the fact that many teens never visit a dentist for regular dental care, and some have never ever been to a dentist at all. The fact is, a child should visit a pediatric dentist as early as possible to nip any potential problems in the bud. For example, an infection dur-

Diabetes—Type 1

It happens without warning. It affects people in all walks of life. And there is nothing you can do to prevent it. This is Type 1 diabetes, a malfunction of the pancreas, an organ of the digestive system, that affects more than a million people in the United States. (See page 212 for details about Type 2 diabetes.) Because it's usually diagnosed in children or young adults, the peak age for diagnosis being fourteen, it is often called juvenile diabetes or early-onset diabetes. The fundamental cause of Type 1 diabetes is that the pancreas—the organ that makes insulin, which is the hormone that helps metabolize sugar—has failed and can no longer make enough insulin to control the level of sugar in your blood. The problem with having high levels of sugar in your body is that it ultimately damages your small blood vessels, which in turn leads to cardiovascular disease, blindness, nerve damage, and kidney damage.

No one knows why somebody gets early-onset diabetes, but several pathways are suspected. One is heredity. Perhaps there is a family predisposition for a gene aberration that causes the pancreas to fail early in life. Viral infections are also suspect; perhaps in the course of fighting off an infection the immune system mistakenly attacks the pancreas and the result is an organ that doesn't work. But whatever the root cause, the bottom line is that your pancreas produces very little or no insulin at all, and you have to supplement this shortfall by injecting yourself with insulin starting early in life.

Juvenile diabetics must learn early on to lead a really healthy lifestyle. You cannot have juvenile diabetes and not take care of yourself. If you take up smoking and drinking, ignoring nutrition and exercise, you won't be in this world for long. But if you maintain a healthy lifestyle and monitor your blood sugar level on a daily basis, which is very important, you will be able to lead a relatively healthy life, even though you will be at risk of developing chronic diseases by your fifties and sixties.

ing pregnancy can leave a child's teeth without the protective enamel they normally have, a situation that demands the attention of a dentist. And to prevent dental deterioration during the "sweet years," dentists recommend that children have their teeth sealed. The sealant is placed on the grooves on the tops of children's teeth to prevent the bacteria and food particles from settling into those grooves. Since they fill in the deep part of the fissure on top of the tooth, the sealant will generally stay in the tooth for years. After that, it's a good idea to visit the dentist twice a year for a good cleaning. Most kids are not exactly conscientious when brushing their teeth, so this serves as a good backup.

The long-term issues of poor dental health are more serious than you might think, and I'm not talking about losing your teeth and being unable to eat. Chronic gingivitis caused by bacteria and cavities as a youth has, in the later years, significant implications for heart disease. How? Gum disease may damage the small blood vessels in the gums, allowing bacteria to enter the bloodstream. The bacteria may then trigger the clumping of platelets, forming blood clots that can block arteries and lead to a heart attack or blocked arteries in the brain, leading to a stroke. In fact, studies show that people with advanced gum disease have from 25 to 100 percent greater risk of heart attack than those without advanced gum disease. Gastric ulcers may also occur as a result of poor dental hygiene; the bacteria *H. pylori,* which has been found in the mucosa of ulcer sufferers, is now known to cause gastric ulcers. So brush your teeth and gums regularly, change your toothbrush often (it's been how many years, you say?), and visit your dentist for that squeaky-clean-teeth feeling.

Turning Obesity on Its Head (Bulimia)

America's obsession with appearance is out of control, and it's having a profound impact on our teenagers. Fifty percent of all teenage girls are practically starving themselves to stay thin. According to one study,

50 percent of teenage girls always skip breakfast and do not know proper eating habits. Fifteen percent would consider taking laxatives or making themselves sick to keep their weight down. What we are talking about here is bulimia.

Bulimia is an illness defined by recurrent episodes of binge eating followed by vomiting or other methods to prevent weight gain. It's more likely to occur in the later teenage years. The bulimic individual is usually of normal weight, unless the bulimia is also accompanied by anorexia, an eating disorder involving severe, chronic weight loss (see "Too Thin (Anorexia)," page 79). Like obesity, bulimia stems from having poor eating habits, getting too little exercise, and living in a world where the media decides whom we should admire. Peer pressure from friends plays a large role in the development of bulimia in girls—you rarely get bulimia in a boy. (In general, boys are not as conscious of their appearance as girls are.) Girls are more mature and more social creatures, which means they are more likely to fall into the trap of needing to fit in with their peers.

Bulimia is a psychological problem with potentially serious health effects. It affects 1 percent of all teenagers. Binge eating followed by vomiting causes a loss of electrolytes (sodium, potassium, and chloride), a loss of nutrients, a loss of fluids, and a loss of body mass. So your body is in a malnourished state, and that impacts your immune system, allowing you to become susceptible to all sorts of viral infections. The continuous vomiting can alter the mechanics of your heart, kidneys, and liver. Earlier I compared obesity to putting fifty gallons of gasoline into a twenty-gallon tank. Bulimia is like putting a dollar of gas in your tank and running on empty all the time. You are always sucking the bottom of the tank, the carburetor is getting full of suds, and you are constantly at risk of running out of gas. Ultimately, the bulimic individual faces the equivalent of stopping in the middle of the highway and having a major accident.

Since bulimics tend to be of average weight, it is difficult to recognize bulimic individuals simply by looking at their appearance, but a careful observer can learn to read the hidden signs of the disease (see "The Hidden Signs of Bulimia," page 78). Recovery from bulimia requires treatment, lifestyle changes, and the resolution of the underlying psychological and social issues that triggered the problem. To identify these issues, solve the problems, and overcome the fears, psychotherapy is an essential ingredient in the treatment of bulimia. Nutritional counseling is also often necessary to restore physical health, and a doctor can prescribe drugs to help reduce the binging and purging of bulimia, as well as treat the depression and anxiety that often accompanies it.

Bulimia is a difficult problem to tackle, because, again, the media has such a significant influence on our lives. Just at the age when teenagers are trying to develop a personal identity and body image, the entertainment industry creates within them a desire to be the most popular, the prettiest, the thinnest. Everything today is targeted to popularity and good looks, especially for teenagers. That is the message the media dishes out every day. When unchecked by parents and a supportive home life, adolescent children exposed to that constant message can end up believing that being thin is what's most important in life and that everything else will follow.

Most girls who are bulimic are also depressed. Why depression? Because they never feel that they have achieved their goal. They never feel popular enough, pretty enough, thin enough. Their ideal body image always lies just over the horizon. It's an illusion with dire consequences.

The Hidden Signs of Bulimia

- Bulimics tend to have low self-esteem and may be depressed.
- They often have difficulty expressing their emotions.
- They seem to consume large amounts of food with no change in weight.
- They have odd eating behaviors and tend to eat alone.
- They are secretive about the time period after eating or have complex lifestyle schedules to make time for their binge-and-purge sessions.
- They are preoccupied with their body image and may wear baggy clothes.
- They have an excessive and rigid exercise routine.
- They have callused or colored finger joints or backs of the hands from jamming their fingers down their throats to induce vomiting.
- They have discolored or decalcified teeth and swollen or bleeding cheeks and gums, caused both by vitamin deficiencies and the stomach acid that comes up with vomit.

Too Thin (Anorexia)

Compared to the bulimic individual, the person with the eating disorder called *anorexia nervosa* is an easy read. Anorexics, as they are known, weigh 85 percent or less of what a normal person of their age and height usually weighs. Anorexics have an absolute fear of becoming fat and, in fact, believe they are fat even though they are very thin. Rather than regurgitating what they eat like bulimics, anorexics simply reduce how much they eat, often to fewer than a thousand calories per day. As a result, their nails, hair, and bones become brittle; their skin may become dry and yellow; and they become depressed and often complain of being cold. In young girls, menstruation is delayed, and in women, menstrual periods stop. Eventually, the lack of nutrition will damage the heart and brain.

Anorexia nervosa predominately affects adolescent girls and young adult women, although it can also occur in men and older women. About 0.5 to 1 percent of females in the United States become anorexic. As with bulimia, treatment for anorexics requires psychotherapy to deal with the underlying emotional issues. The complications associated with anorexia are reversible once their weight is restored. A weight gain of one to three pounds a week is considered safe. Obviously, the sooner the problem is recognized and treated, the better.

Depression

Depression among children is a serious problem. One out of every twenty adolescents suffers from clinical depression. When depression begins during the teenage years, the risks are significant, interrupting both learning and the development of those parts of the brain where decisions are made. And among depressed teens, suicide is a significant risk. Suicide is responsible for more than 10 percent of the deaths in the fifteen-to-nineteen age group.

There are many reasons for depression. Suffering loss such as the death of a parent or a friend, or experiencing extreme trauma can trigger depression, of course. Other well-known links to childhood depression include physical and sexual abuse, neglect, inappropriate criticism, conflict in the family, divorce, addiction in the family, violence in the family, racism, and poverty. Some depression may be genetic at core and be caused by a chemical imbalance in the brain. But even then, the genetic predisposition must be triggered by a trauma or stressful event of some sort.

The most troubling aspect of depression in children is that it often goes undiagnosed. Parents must be on the lookout for signs of depression. Sometimes the signs are obvious. The child always seems sad, lacks energy, and has no interest in activities he or she once considered fun. Other signs may include a sudden change in sleeping or eating habits—either sleeping too much or too little, or eating too much or too little. The child may also display increased irritability, anger, or hostility. He or she may not want to go to school, may have falling grades, may have difficulty getting along with others, or may exhibit low self-esteem.

Depression is a persistent condition; it's more than just having the "blues" now and then. But if you feel that your child is truly depressed, don't brush it off, thinking that it will go away by itself. Deal with it immediately.

The most important thing parents must do with a depressed child is to break the barrier of communication. Begin by telling your child that you care about how he or she feels. I realize that telling a child how you feel about him or her can be very difficult. But to me, the words "I love you" are absolutely fundamental in establishing a good relationship with your child. It's incredibly important for parents to let their children know how they feel, to use the words "I love you; I want you to feel better." Be sure your child knows that you are concerned. If I, as a doctor, attempt to treat depression by saying, "Take this pill and go home," I won't have accomplished anything. It's like treating a fever with Tylenol; the fever will go down but if I haven't found out what caused the fever, I haven't rendered a cure. It's the same with depression. You need to know where it's coming from to be able to treat it.

Try to find out why it is that your child feels unenergetic, why he or she is moping around all day; but don't make the mistake of asking straight out, "Why are you sad all the time?" If you do, you won't get a coherent answer. It's better to deal with the half-full part of the glass rather than the half-empty part. In other words, ask your child what he or she is into lately, what gets the mojo working. You must express interest in what he or she is doing. And you have to learn to read between the lines of any response you get.

Kids are sometimes more sensitive to their parents' feelings than we think. They can sense when their parents are worried, when their parents are not getting along, when their parents are having trouble at work, and even when the parents themselves are depressed. So it is fundamental for parents to be open about their own feelings as well. Emotions are the beauty of our soul, and if we don't share them, if we don't teach our children how to share them, then and once again we fall into that trap of not leading by example. You cannot expect a child to talk to you about his or her feelings when you don't express your own feelings. It's okay to tell a child, "Look, I've got problems, but don't worry. I'm strong. I know that life is not perfect, and I'll get through it." Once you share your feelings, maybe your child will begin sharing his or her feelings with you. At that point, one of the first messages you should get across to the depressed child is that if he or she shares whatever it is that is causing the sadness, you can help him or her get through it. That will give the child hope.

In more severe cases, when you feel that professional help is needed, be sure to involve the child in this decision. Don't suddenly take your child to your primary care doctor, the pediatrician, or a mental health specialist. That action will simply label your child as "the problem," and nothing positive will be gained. There is no quick fix to depression. Your child must be involved in any solution that's needed to resolve the depression. If you feel a doctor is needed, before you make that appointment, explain to your child that the doctor, psychologist, or mental health worker is a fundamental part of the healing process. You might share your own personal experience, how such people have helped you, or cite any example you know of that might be of help in getting the child to understand how doctors are there to help us, whatever our problems may be.

The first step in the treatment of depression must address any environmental or family problems. If the child is being sexually abused, for instance, obviously the child cannot continue to have contact with the abuser. Any poor relationships with parents, siblings, teachers, and friends must be repaired, as a supportive social network prevents the isolation and loneliness that often leads to or exacerbates depression. If there are adults in the family who are depressed, their depression must also be addressed and treated. In fact, a new study has found that treating a mother's depression can help prevent depression and anxiety disorders in her children.

There are many ways other than medication to treat depression. Exercise and daily walks have both proven to be excellent therapy for children as well as adults. Meditation, prayer, relaxation, and yoga are also very effective. Two big-ticket items in the arsenal of simple treatments for depression are nature and pets. Studies have found that the more time you spend outdoors with nature, the less depressed you tend to be. Also true is that families with pets are families with a lower incidence of childhood depression.

Food can also play an important role in improving moods and fighting depression. The foods you eat should provide a continuous supply of the nutrients you need to keep your brain chemically balanced. Deficiencies of vitamin B_{12}, vitamin B_6, vitamin C, and folic acid have all been linked with depression. Research has also confirmed the antidepressant-like effects of omega-3 fatty acids, which are found in cold-water fish like sardines, tuna, and Atlantic salmon, and some plant sources such as canola oil and walnuts. Apparently uridine, a compound found in sugar beets and molasses, has similar antidepressant effects. On the other hand, you want to avoid simple carbohydrates such as candy and sugar; these foods can cause quick highs and lows that may actually contribute to depression.

Depression can also be controlled with medication. But this is a difficult issue: should children and adolescents be given antidepressants? The problem is that the information available for treating depressed children with antidepressants can be both confusing and frightening. Studies indicate that antidepressants are not always effective in improving depression in children and adolescents. Debate also continues on the optimal length of treatment. And some studies have shown that the use of antidepressants may increase the risk of suicidal thoughts and behaviors.

But when psychotherapy doesn't help, or when children are having serious depression-related difficulties functioning at home and school, antidepressants may be the only alternative. The bottom line is that antidepressants are potent drugs that should be avoided unless absolutely necessary, and then should be used only under the supervision of a well-trained child psychiatrist.

Once a child or adolescent starts on an antidepressant, the FDA recommends the following frequency of doctor visits:

- Once a week for four weeks
- Every two weeks for the next month
- At the end of the twelfth week taking the drug
- More often if problems or questions arise

Depressingly Wrong

MYTH: It's normal for teenagers to be moody. It eventually just goes away.

FACT: Depression is more than just being moody. It can affect people at any age.

MYTH: A kid who really needs help will ask for it.

FACT: Depression interferes with a person's ability or desire to get help. If a friend is depressed, tell an adult. That's not betraying a trust; in fact, you might be saving a life.

MYTH: A person who talks about suicide doesn't do it.

FACT: Suicidal thoughts, remarks, or attempts are always serious. Get help for someone talking about suicide immediately.

MYTH: Talking about depression only makes it worse.

FACT: Talking about your feelings is the first step toward beating depression. A depressed person needs someone to talk to for support and encouragement.

MYTH: Few teenagers actually commit suicide.

FACT: About two thousand teens kill themselves every year in the United States. It is the leading cause of death among teenagers. Five of every twenty-five teenagers have seriously considered suicide, and two of those are likely to have tried to kill themselves in the past year.

We must remember that depression itself can be a dangerous disorder, and that antidepressants, if used properly, can save lives.

Substance Abuse

The teenage years are without a doubt the most exciting time of life. There is a Teflon quality to the teenage years, a belief that nothing can affect them. Unfortunately, teenagers often fail to link their actions to consequences. As a result, this period of experimentation and growing up can be quite a dangerous time. Data shows that more and more teenagers today are using alcohol as well as legal and illegal drugs than at any time in history. And when individuals start drinking alcohol and smoking early in their teenage years, they are more likely to use illicit drugs in their later years.

There are many reasons why teenagers exhibit this type of behavior. Curiosity is one, stress reduction another, but using drugs can also make them feel good or make them feel grown up. The risk of teenage substance abuse also has to do with family history. Teens who have a parent who is a substance abuser tend to be substance abuses, too. If there's a strong history of depression in a family, substance abuse can be a problem for the teenagers in that family. For teens who have issues of low self-esteem because their home environment fails to reinforce positive behaviors, substance abuse may be a consequence.

Teenagers are more likely to abuse alcohol than any other drug. Why? Because it's so easily obtained at home. They see their parents do it, and they think, *Well, if they do it, it's okay for me to do it.* And certainly most parents do not educate their children about alcohol consumption and the difference between proper use and abuse. Teenagers will also abuse other products easily available in the house—popping both prescription and over-the-counter medications such as diet and sleeping pills, as well as sniffing glues, solvents, and aerosols.

Among illegal drugs, marijuana is very prevalent among teenagers today. School surveys have shown that children as young as thirteen are using marijuana, so this is clearly a major problem. Other illegal drugs available to teenagers include cocaine, crack, speed, heroin, and the club

Drinking and Driving
(d + d = D?)

Car accidents continue to be the lead-ing cause of death for fifteen- to twenty-year-olds. Three thousand to four thousand teenagers are killed in car crashes each year, and more than three hundred thousand are injured. A third of those killed had been drinking, and three-quarters of them were not wearing safety belts. Almost three-quarters of teens in the tenth grade—usually the year they begin to drive—say they drink alcohol. Parents need to talk to their teens about slowing down, buckling up, and never, ever driving under the influence of alcohol.

drug Ecstasy. The use of any of these drugs can put teenagers in terrible danger, for everything from car accidents to unprotected sex to suicide. And a teenage lifestyle that features drugs, precocious sex, and other risky behaviors also usually includes seri-ous violence. Violence itself is a serious problem with American teenagers. About 30 to 40 percent of all male youths and 15 to 30 percent of all female youths report having committed a serious violent offense by age seventeen. This peaks at about age sixteen and drops off dramatically by age twenty. For intervention to succeed, parents must confront not only the violent behavior of these teenagers but their risky lifestyles as well.

Parents must learn to heed the warning signs of substance abuse. The physical signs include fatigue, coughing, and glassy eyes. The emotional signs in-clude irritability, mood changes, lack of responsible behavior, and depression. Many teenage substance abusers become disin-terested in schoolwork and activities and, ultimately, end up with social problems by hanging out with the wrong crowd.

Parents should try to deal with substance abuse by directly confronting the issue. There is no easy solution to dealing with teenagers who are abusing drugs. But clearly, the parents must try to get to the root of the problem. A family physician can test for substance abuse, but often a men-tal health professional will need to be involved in order to break the im-passe of communication. Alcohol abuse usually requires attendance at a rehabilitation center, and, afterward, parents must keep a dialogue open with their teenagers in order to prevent a relapse. The bottom line is that early recognition and early treatment are the keys to helping teenagers with substance abuse problems.

Cigarette Smoking

Cigarettes are also drugs; nicotine is highly addictive and a major public health problem. Some 3 million U.S. teenagers smoke. And about three thousand more teenagers start smoking every day, a third of whom will eventually die prematurely of a smoking-related disease. In fact, smoking is the main cause of lung cancer and heart disease in this country. And the saddest thing about the death and disease caused by cigarette smoking is that it is *preventable.*

Teenagers begin smoking for many reasons. Usually it's because their parents smoke, or their siblings smoke, or their friends smoke. Stress also leads to smoking, as does poor self-esteem. Girls tend to smoke as a way of

Corporate Responsibility

After ten years of steady decline, it seems that smoking trends are not decreasing as fast as we might have expected. Why—after the amount of publicity against smoking, the creation of no-smoking zones, and a decrease in the number of adults smoking—are the statistics not improving? Most teens surveyed today say that "peer pressure and fitting in" were primarily responsible for their picking up the habit. But what about the tobacco companies? They keep coming up with cool stuff like flavored cigarettes. I wonder to whom the tobacco companies are marketing those—my uncle Joe, the wholesale butcher, or the kid down the block?

As I noted earlier, 50 percent of all teenage girls are practically starving themselves to stay thin. American's obsession with appearance is out of control. You think the media could be responsible for that, too? You bet they are.

So where do we go from here? I guess more parental involvement. That seems to be the response I get whenever I bring up the subject of corporate responsibility. There are those who say it is the parents, and only the parents, who are responsible for making sure their children eat right, don't smoke, and don't drink. Look, I know firsthand how challenging parenting can be. We need a little help! Society in general needs to get involved to help protect our future generations. So how about it? How about some corporate responsibility?

dealing with poor academic performance, and some begin to smoke as a way of controlling their weight.

Teenagers who smoke also tend to engage in more risky behaviors. They get into more fights, tend to carry weapons, have sex at an earlier age, fail to wear seat belts in a car, and tend to use illegal drugs later on. Statistics show that most adult smokers began smoking before the age of eighteen. And the earlier individuals start smoking, the greater their risk for developing major diseases like lung cancer and heart disease, and the harder it is for them to quit.

How can we stop this problem? Simple. Parents must be role models. If you have teenagers or young children at home and you smoke, then you are a walking and talking billboard for the cigarette companies. If you truly believe that smoking is bad, then don't smoke yourself, and forbid smoking in your home—both for the other residents of your house and anyone who visits. Make sure that tobacco education is integrated in the curriculum of the school your teen attends. Don't let little children have toys or candies that emulate smoking in any way, shape, or form, like candy cigarettes. If you have a teenager who has already started smoking, help him or her stop. Provide educational materials and create an environment that encourages quitting. If you smoke yourself and your teenager picks up the habit, think of it as the perfect time for both of you to quit together. One of the most difficult things for an adult to do is to quit smoking. If you have a child who has picked up the habit, use that as a motivator to stop smoking yourself.

Sexually Transmitted Diseases (STDs)

Teenagers and sexuality—it's a volatile mix and an inevitable fact of life. Hormones are flowing, peer pressure is on the rise, media is fueling the sexual fires, and sex education in the United States is limited at best. Two-thirds of American high-school students have had sex by their senior year.

As a result, sexually transmitted diseases (STDs)—those infections that spread during vaginal, anal, and oral sex—are very common in teenagers. One out of four sexually active teenagers—the age group with the highest rates of sexually transmitted diseases in this country—has a sexually transmitted disease. The most common sexually transmitted diseases are trichomoniasis, genital warts, chlamydia, gonorrhea, and herpes. Less common are syphilis and HIV. Most teenagers with an STD don't even know they have it because STDs often don't produce any symptoms. When left untreated in teenagers, STDs can mean chronic pain in the young adult years as well as infertility, cancers, and other diseases. Almost all STDs have cures, so early treatment can help prevent permanent damage. Teenagers living anywhere in the United States can get tested and treated for STDs confidentially, that is, without a parent or guardian's knowledge.

Trichomoniasis, or trichomonas, is one of the most common sexually transmitted diseases in teenagers. It is caused by a parasite that lives in the female vagina or in the male urethra. Infected females may have a yellowish, greenish vaginal discharge and significant vaginal irritation. Infected males may have burning upon urination. But half of the females who contract trichomonas have no symptoms, and males almost never do. Trichomonas is very easy for a doctor to diagnose; an examination of the discharge under the microscope will reveal the culprit. And with medication, it's 100 percent curable.

Chlamydia is even more of a stealth sexual disease than trichomonas. Symptoms, if they show up at all, develop about a week after intercourse. Females may experience a discharge, pain upon urination, dull abdominal pain, nausea, or some vaginal spotting. But 90 percent of women with chlamydia do not know that they have it. Males with chlamydia may have a watery drip from their penis, but that's very rare; most males have no symptoms at all. A doctor can diagnose the disease by testing the urethral, or cervical, discharge. Treatment with simple antibiotics is very effective. The problem with chlamydia, because it rarely displays symptoms, is that untreated females may develop a condition called pelvic inflammatory disease, or PID. In PID the uterus, ovaries, and especially the fallopian tubes get so inflamed and scarred from the chronic infection that the woman may end up unable to conceive. Even in some males, chlamydia, when left untreated, can ultimately damage the sperm passageway and also lead to male sterility. If a pregnant woman delivers with an active chlamydia infection, the baby can develop pneumonia or eye infections.

Gonorrhea goes by many names, including the clap or the drip. Symptoms develop anywhere between two to twenty-one days after exposure. Females will experience a thick yellow or green discharge, accompanied by burning upon urination, abdominal pain or tenderness, and an abnormal menstrual period. Males may also experience a burning upon urination and a thick yellow drip from their penis. A test of the urine or the secretion, from either the vagina, the cervix, or the penis, confirms the diagnosis. Treatment with antibiotics is very effective and 100 percent safe. But again, when left untreated, gonorrhea will cause infertility, as well as chronic joint pain, a gonorrheal type of arthritis, and damage to the eyes and heart.

Herpes, also known as HSV (herpes simplex virus), is a viral infection that manifests within two to thirty days after having sex. Males and females get similar flulike symptoms—fever, aches, and fatigue—as well as very painful blisters on the genitals, or in the mouth in the case of oral sex. The blisters can last anywhere between one and three weeks. An examination of the lesions is usually sufficient to confirm the diagnosis of herpes. Herpes is very easily transmitted, and once you get it, the virus stays with you for the rest of your life. There is really no treatment for herpes because nothing kills the virus. But some drugs are effective in reducing the frequency and duration of outbreaks, which tend to diminish over time anyway (see "The Two Herpes," page 93).

Human papilloma virus, or HPV, is *the* most common sexually transmitted disease. Most infections don't produce any symptoms, and HPV infections can clear up on their own; if the virus persists, however, it may lead to genital warts, either in the vulva or on the penis. One indirect problem associated with HPV is that it can alter the results of the Pap smear, the cancer test of the female genital tract. Some kinds of HPVs have been strongly associated with cervical cancer, which is why doctors need to identify the specific type of HPV; after diagnosis doctors will treat the affected area by either freezing, by applying chemicals, or by surgically removing it to prevent its transformation into a cancerous lesion. In 2006, the FDA approved a vaccine, called Gardasil, that guards against 70 percent of cervical cancers and 90 percent of genital warts caused by HPV. The Advisory Committee on Immunization Practices (ACIP) has recommended that girls as young as eleven routinely get the new vaccine in hopes of protecting them before they become sexually active. (For more on Gardasil, see page 151.)

Syphilis is not the devastating sexually transmitted disease it once was because there's now a golden bullet for it: penicillin—and only penicillin—can cure it completely. But treating syphilis early, before the disease, which affects both men and women similarly, progresses to its serious second or third stages, is important. In the first stage of syphilis, reddish chancre sores may appear on the genitals, mouth, or anus one to twelve weeks after sexual contact. In the second stage, which takes place one to six months after contact, a rash may appear on the chest, back, arms, and legs, accompanied by a fever, sore throat, and enlarged lymph nodes. These symptoms may come and go. The third stage of syphilis, three years or more after contact, produces ulcers on the skin and internal organs, as well as arthritis and sensory dysfunction, and perhaps damage to the heart, spinal cord, and brain. The diagnosis of syphilis is made through a physical exam and blood test.

HIV is a sexually transmitted disease that can also be acquired by sharing intravenous needles and by exposure to infected body fluids like blood or semen. Most people with HIV have no symptoms, especially in the early stages of the disease. Symptoms can appear several months after HIV exposure, starting with a recurrent fever, unexplained weight loss, swollen lymph glands, fatigue, diarrhea, loss of appetite, and white spots or blemishes in the mouth. As HIV progresses, it causes extensive immune system damage, which is called AIDS, or acquired immune deficiency syndrome. Though there is no cure for HIV, medical therapy can control the virus and prolong the life of infected individuals.

Perhaps the most frightening thing about many STDs is that individuals can contract them without having any symptoms to alert them that they're actually infected. If symptoms do show up, most people will then seek treatment for them. But what about people who are infected and don't have any symptoms? STDs do not go away without treatment, even if the symptoms themselves disappear.

So who's telling teenagers about these diseases? If you took a survey of sixteen- or eighteen-year-olds and asked them, "What's chlamydia?," most of them would look at you as if you had three heads. They have no idea what it is. Don't assume your teenager knows about STDs. And don't depend on the sex-education class at school to tell them, assuming your local school even offers one. Less than half the states require schools to provide sex education, even though more than 90 percent of Americans favor some type of sex education in school. (The debate is now over what ex-

The Two Herpes

There are two types of herpes simplex virus. One has a social stigma attached to it; the other doesn't. HSV-1 is the usual cause of cold sores. HSV-2 is the usual cause of genital herpes. About one-third of Americans have HSV-1, having acquired it when they were children. Only one-quarter of Americans have HSV-2, which is usually acquired as teenagers or adults. But in reality, the differences between the two are not as great as their wildly different public perceptions.

HSV-1 and HSV-2 are virtually identical under a microscope. Both infect the mucosal surfaces, either the mouth or the genitals, before establishing themselves in the nervous system. Two-thirds of people infected with either virus show few or no symptoms. HSV-1 tends to establish itself in a collection of nerve cells near the ear, called the trigeminal ganglion, before manifesting on the lower lip or face. HSV-2 tends to establish itself at a location at the base of the spine, called the sacral ganglion, before appearing in the genital area. But actually both types can reside in, and infect, either or both parts of the body.

While HSV-1 is commonly viewed as a mild infection that is bothersome but not dangerous, HSV-2 is perceived as a painful and dangerous infection that affects only very sexually active people. In reality, each one may lead to rare but dangerous complications. HSV-1 can on occasion affect the eyes and cause blindness, or it can spread to the brain and cause herpes encephalitis, a dangerous infection that can lead to death. HSV-2, on the other hand, is the most common cause of neonatal herpes, a rare but dangerous infection in newborns.

actly should be taught, not over whether it should or shouldn't be taught.) Some states may teach teens about HIV/AIDS but not about any other STD or about how to prevent pregnancy. So if you haven't spoken to your children about sex, all they are likely to know about it is what they've see in the media and what they've learned from their peers. In other words, they probably know next to nothing about STDs.

The only way to really prevent sexually transmitted disease is by educating your children, having a healthy dialogue about sex. It's best to start talking about sex in the preteen years, or the middle-school years, but it's never too late to talk about sex and sexually transmitted diseases. Some kids—depending on their age, gender, and level of maturity—may be very inquisitive about sexual education by the time they're nine or ten, while others won't be interested in the subject until some years later. You will need to read the clues your children provide to determine when they are most likely to feel comfortable discussing the subject.

When you do talk to your children about sex, put them in charge of the conversation. This is their conversation, not yours, and you'll have a better interaction that way. Ask your teenagers what they already know about sexually transmitted diseases. Ask them what they think about sexual scenarios on television or in movies when they see one. Do they understand what is happening? Build a dialogue in this way. Encourage your children to raise any fears or concerns they may have; if you provide them with the appropriate tools, they're going to be better prepared later to decide not to have intercourse when they really don't want to. And at the end of the day, you can bring home the fundamental point that the only *sure* way to remain free from sexually transmitted disease is not to engage in sex or other intimate contact with anyone outside of a monogamous relationship such as marriage.

The Kissing Disease—Mononucleosis

Despite its reputation as "the kissing disease," mononucleosis is not a sexually transmitted disease. Mono, as it's also known, got tagged with the kissing moniker because it often appears around the dating age and because it can, in fact, be transmitted through a kiss. But the disease can also be spread by sharing a drinking glass or eating utensils, or by being on the wrong end of a sneeze or a cough. That said, however, mono is not highly contagious.

The disease, which is most common among adolescents, often sneaks up on individuals. At first it may seem like just another bad sore throat and fever, but eventually the fatigue that accompanies mono identifies it as probably being infectious mononucleosis. The disease gets its formal name from the fact that there is a significant increase in the body in the number of white blood cells of a certain kind, those known as mononuclear leukocytes, which have a one-lobed nucleus. Normally these make up about one-third of all white blood cells. But in mono, they can account for one-half or more of the white blood cells present.

The majority of cases of mono are caused by the Epstein-Barr virus (EBV), which produces a fever and makes the glands in the body swell up, though the cytomegalovirus (CMV) can produce a similar illness that's characterized by less sore-throat pain. Most people in the world have been infected with the EBV virus by the age of thirty-five and have developed immunity to it. The few who do develop symptoms of the disease usually experience fatigue, weakness, swollen lymph glands in the neck and armpits, fever, and sore throat for weeks or months. There are several ways to diagnose the disease, including the monospot test, which checks for the presence of EBV in the blood.

Most doctors treating mono recommend bed rest, plenty of liquids, and a healthy diet, if that's not already standard operating procedure. If the mono is not treated in time, if the immune system is not allowed to recuperate, a number of complications may occur. Because mono is a dis-

For Women Only—
The First Gynecological Examination

For many young women, the first visit to a gynecologist is often their first adult encounter with a physician. There is often a long hiatus between their last visit to a pediatrician during their teenage years and their first visit to a doctor as a young adult. When a woman is college bound, or in college, she may need to see a doctor because she's now sexually active and needs contraception, or because she develops a common vaginal condition, like vaginitis or a urinary tract infection. A primary care physician can conduct the gynecological exam if no gynecologist is available.

It's very important that a young woman's first encounter with a gynecologist not be traumatic. I think young women should see their gynecologist for the first time by the age of eighteen or so; it's essential that they learn their pelvic organ status, and begin to develop a health portfolio, especially if they're thinking of having children one day.

During the gynecological examination, a doctor will perform a physical exam of the vaginal area, first by paying attention to the outside anatomy to make sure that it's well developed. Next, the doctor will use a speculum, or polished plate used as a reflector, to inspect the cervix and the vaginal walls. Then, employing something similar to a Q-tip, the doctor will scrape from the cervix some tissue that will later be tested for precancerous and cancerous cells; this is called a Pap test, or Pap smear. The Pap test is designed primarily to detect cervical cancer, which is treatable if found early, but it can also identify hundreds of other minor problems, such as inflammation and the presence of HPV, the human papilloma virus.

The doctor will also examine the patient's breasts for lumps and other changes. Not only will this exam detect lumps or abnormalities, but it should serve as a perfect opportunity, in the first few gynecological visits, for a young woman to learn how to do a breast self-examination. Often the breast self-exam is what alerts a woman to a potential problem, so it's important that she become familiar with her anatomy at an early age to be able to detect any changes that may occur later on.

ease of the body's glands or lymph system, the spleen, which filters the blood, may become enlarged and rupture; the liver can also become enlarged, resulting in a jaundice similar to that produced by hepatitis; anemia, which is a low red blood cell count, can occur; and an inflammation of the meniges, which is the covering of the brain, can develop. There's also some evidence to suggest a link between mononucleosis and the development of multiple sclerosis, a muscle weakness of unknown cause characterized by degenerative lesions in the brain. Other types of chronic diseases that can result from chronic mononucleosis are Bell's palsy and Guillain-Barré syndrome, two neurological muscle diseases. Fatalities are very rare, but mono may not let go easily—relapses do occur in a small percentage of people, particularly in those who fail to properly treat the disease when it first strikes.

Test Checklist for this Decade

	Check BMI
	First gynecological exam (girls at eighteen or when sexually active)
	STDs/HIV tests (when sexually active)
	Physical (yearly)
	Tetanus booster (every ten years)
	Vaccinations updated
	Dental cleaning (yearly)
	Vision and hearing tests (every three years)
	Skin check (every three months)
	Meningitis vaccine (for college students)

Welcome to the Real World

(The Third Decade: Ages 20 to 29)

These are years of profound change. Detached from the parental lifeline, you seek both identity and intimacy. You are at your peak of physical health and fitness and at the height of your cognitive abilities. Use them wisely.

3

What a change a few years can make. In this decade young people make their transition to adulthood. While their bodies may still gain a bit more height and muscle at the beginning of this decade, and their brain is still increasing in size and weight, most individuals in their early twenties have completed their education, joined the workforce, established their own household, and now bear the legal rights, responsibilities, and roles of an adult in this society. By the time people reach their mid-twenties, about eight out of ten no longer live at home, four out of ten are married, and more than nine out of ten males and eight out of ten females have a job. After peaking between ages nineteen and twenty-one, alcohol, marijuana, and other substance use starts to decline during this decade, as does the tendency to commit serious violence. Much of this improved behavior can be attributed to having a stable relationship and a stable job, even if that job involves looking at a computer screen most of the day.

Geek Lifestyle

You don't have to be a certified geek to be troubled by the consequences of the computer-intense lifestyle so common among many energetic young people today. Why? To begin with, there's more than a little bit of geek in all of us at this point. Just count the number of little gadgets and gizmos you depend on every day. Cell phone? BlackBerry? iPod? And, most crucially, how many of you spend hours a day in front of a computer? Welcome to the club. The trademarks of the geek lifestyle are recurrent headaches, back pain, and sleeping problems.

Those headaches are likely the product of having poor sitting posture, positioning the screen improperly, trying to read too small a font, or using a screen that's either too bright or too dark. It could also come from drinking too much coffee or soft drinks and too little water. Proper eye care can also minimize computer-related headaches. Don't wear eyeglasses stronger than you need. Don't forget to blink when staring at your monitor. And remember to shift your gaze regularly from the computer screen to something in the distance—a car, a building, or a cloud—to relieve eye fatigue.

Poor posture and an incorrectly positioned chair and monitor are major contributors to back pain. Adjust the chair height so that your thighs are parallel to the floor and your feet are flat on the floor. Adjust the back support so that your back is perfectly perpendicular to the floor, and be sure to sit all the way back in the chair. Adjust the keyboard so that your forearms are parallel to the floor. And adjust the display or monitor height so that it's about an arm's length away from your eyes and the top of it is at or just below your eye level. Also, every half hour or so, take a break from the keyboard and stretch your arms, hands, neck, and back. And since weak abdominal muscles can also contribute to lower back pain, you should do something to strengthen your back—abdominal crunches at the gym, perhaps, or swimming, or yoga. All these activities will help reduce back pain.

Then there are the sleeping problems, usually insomnia and altered sleep patterns. Are you working late into the night and trying to catch up on your sleep during the day? Are you having trouble falling asleep? Are you waking up in the middle of the night and turning on a laptop or watching TV? The solution involves making sleep a regular habit again. Don't go to bed unless you're tired. Don't watch TV or work in bed. The bed is for sleeping (and sex). If you don't fall asleep in fifteen minutes or so, get up and read a book or listen to music. Whatever you do, don't go back to work. And try to go to bed and wake up at the same time day after day.

Debilitating Headaches

There are headaches, and then there are *migraine* headaches. Any headache can make you miserable, but a migraine can be excruciating. In fact, the most severe migraine headaches can just about bring you to your knees.

More than 28 million Americans suffer from migraine headaches. Their frequency and severity varies from person to person, but they strike women three times more often than men. And if there is a history of migraine in your family, there is an 80 percent chance you will have them as well.

Most people who suffer from migraines will have a first attack by the age of thirty. Often they begin in childhood and then increase in frequency in adolescence. The condition usually continues through the thirties and forties, but attacks tend to decrease in frequency and severity with age, and they are rare after age fifty.

Some people with these painful headaches will experience a variety of visual symptoms—such as flashing lights, blind spots, or zigzag patterns—either before or during the headaches themselves. Migraines make many people feel nauseous or light-headed. Vomiting and an extreme sensitivity to light and sound are other common symptoms. A migraine can incapacitate you for hours or even days.

While there is no cure for migraines and the exact cause of migraines is not known, they are now viewed as a vascular and inflammatory problem, so the new therapies being developed for migraine sufferers are focusing on these two pathways. Not long ago aspirin was the sole remedy for migraines, but today there are medications that can help reduce the frequency of migraine headaches and stop the pain once it has started. Severe cases are now treated with triptans, a class of drugs specifically developed to treat migraines. These drugs normally provide relief within fifteen minutes to two hours in most people.

Preventive medication is available for serious migraine suffers, though they do not eliminate the migraines completely. The beta-blockers used to treat high blood pressure and coronary artery disease can reduce the frequency and severity of migraines, and certain antidepressants can also help prevent migraines. It's important for migraine sufferers to avoid certain triggers, such as smoking, or certain foods or smells that may have triggered their headaches in the past. Birth control pills and other sources of estrogen may also trigger or make the headaches worse if you are a woman. Regular aerobic exercise is highly recommended to reduce tension and to help prevent migraines.

Baby Time—or Not

The twenties are an ideal time to have a child; the body is in an ideal state for it (if you are considering getting pregnant, read the preface to this book, which deals with those crucial nine months). But for some women, though the body may be ready, the mind is not. Perhaps you are pursuing a career that doesn't leave time for child rearing and are waiting until your thirties, which certainly is a popular option these days. If so, you may be looking for a way to prevent pregnancy.

The more we understand our bodies and how they work, the better choices we can make regarding our health. This is particularly true when it comes to contraception. Since men usually play a passive role when it comes to contraception, women have had to carry the burden of responsibility for birth control. So I think that the choice of birth control methods is one that a woman needs to make on her own. That said, I think it's important for couples to talk about their contraception choices, and men should be a little more sensitive to everything that women have to do to avoid a pregnancy.

The choice of contraceptive methods has never been greater than it is today, but, as always, that choice should be based on the woman's health, the frequency of sexual activity, the number of sexual partners, and the desire to have children in the future. Each of the various methods available involves some risks that must be considered.

The simplest and most obvious type of birth control is the barrier method, and the most popular type of barrier method for birth control is the latex or polyurethane *condom*, which exists for both men and women. The condom works by preventing the sperm from reaching the egg. Condoms will fail eleven times out of a hundred and may cause latex allergy, irritation, and vaginitis. On the other hand, condoms happen to be one of the best methods of preventing sexually transmitted diseases such as chlamydia, syphilis, gonorrhea, HIV, and hepatitis.

Another type of barrier method is the *diaphragm*, which is a dome-shaped rubber device that a woman places inside the vagina, usually accompanied with a spermicidal cream, which kills the sperm. The diaphragm will fail seventeen times out of a hundred and counts among its side effects irritation, discomfort, urinary tract infection, and, in rare cases, toxic shock syndrome, especially when the diaphragm is not removed.

Another barrier method is the *cervical cap*, a diaphragm-like device. The cap is placed inside the cervix by a gynecologist, often with great difficulty. Its side effects and failure rates are similar to those of the diaphragm.

Several other birth control methods use a spermicidal cream. One is the *sponge*, a disk-shaped polyurethane device that is easily inserted at the time of intercourse and contains a spermicidal cream called nonoxynol-9. It has a good pregnancy prevention rate, failing only fourteen times in a hundred.

Some women use a *spermicide,* nonoxynol-9, alone, in foam, jelly, or suppository form. Spermicides sometimes cause irritations and allergies, and they have a very poor efficacy rate, failing fifty out of a hundred times.

The *oral contraceptive pill* is probably the most popular method of birth control, probably because it's easy to use and very effective. First introduced in the 1960s, the Pill is a combination of estrogen and progestin hormones that essentially tell the body not to ovulate or release an egg from the ovaries. The Pill today contains very small quantities of both estrogen and progesterone, and it's taken on a daily basis so that the body doesn't get exposed to excessive amounts of the hormones at one time. The pill is very effective, with only two failures in a hundred. The problem is that the Pill does not prevent sexually transmitted diseases, and it can cause menstrual irregularities and stroke. The standard Pill is not recommended for women who are breast-feeding, though it is safe to take a progestin-only birth control pill while breast-feeding (see "The Pill and Breast Cancer?," page 108).

Requiring even less attention than the pill is the *hormone patch,* Ortho Evra. The patch is worn on the abdomen or thigh, where progestin and estrogen are released and then absorbed by the skin. The problem with the patch is that it has been linked to high hormone levels and significant reports of strokes in young women. Just like with the Pill, anyone who has a family history of stroke, is a smoker, or is known to have a heart disorder should probably not use these types of devices.

Another hormone-based device is the vaginal *contraceptive ring,* called the NuvaRing. This two-inch flexible ring, when placed in the vagina, releases progesterone and estrogen. It is very effective, resulting in only one to two pregnancies per hundred.

Perhaps the most effective of all forms of contraception is the *hormone injection,* Depo Provera, which is essentially a shot of progestin that interferes with ovulation. An injection is needed every three months. The side effects include irregular bleeding, weight gain, and headaches. But it is incredibly effective in preventing pregnancy, with fewer than one failure per one hundred.

The *intrauterine device* is better known as the IUD, or the Coil. This method was very popular in the early 1970s and is still used in Europe today. The IUD is a copper T-shaped device inserted by a doctor inside the uterus to prevent the implantation of the egg. Unfortunately, it causes a lot of cramping and heavy bleeding. And in many cases this foreign body leads to the formation of pelvic inflammatory disease, an infection of the uterus and tubes that can cause infertility problems. An IUD is recommended only for women in monogamous relationships because the device acts as a highway for sexually transmitted diseases.

Periodic abstinence is perhaps the oldest known method of birth control. It involves deliberately refraining from having intercourse during the period of ovulation. It's actually quite effective when compared to some other methods, with a failure rate of about twenty per one hundred. But it's critical that women practicing abstinence as a form of birth control be *very* familiar with how the body functions. They have to know exactly when they're menstruating and when they're ovulating. For those who choose this option, each member of the couple must become very familiar with all the different stages of ovulation.

The most permanent method of birth control is *sterilization.* In the male, the procedure is called a *vasectomy* and involves cutting the tubes that connect the testicles, where the sperm is produced, to the prostate, thereby preventing the sperm from entering the semen. In the female, the procedure is called a *tubal ligation,* better known as having one's "tubes tied," and involves closing the fallopian tubes, thereby preventing eggs from traveling down into the uterus where they can be fertilized. Sterilization is highly effective in preventing pregnancy, with fewer than one failure in a hundred. Though these procedures may be reversible, the choice of sterilization should be well thought out and discussed with your doctor.

The only available postcoital contraception option is known as *Plan B,* or the morning-after pill. Introduced in the late 1990s, this is an emergency contraception tool that must be taken within seventy-two hours of engaging in unprotected sex. It should *not* be used routinely because it involves taking pills with high quantities of progesterone, or progesterone with estrogen. The morning-after pill helps reduce the chance of a pregnancy by 80 percent for a single act of unprotected sex. But there are significant side effects involved, including nausea, vomiting, and abdominal pain.

The Pill and Breast Cancer?

You have no doubt heard the stories about a possible link between birth control pills and breast cancer. (See Breast Cancer, page 173.) Whether or not this link is real is difficult to determine, however, since the results from various studies are conflicting. Yes, the more hormones you put into your body, the greater your risk of getting breast cancer. But if you're on birth control pills for short periods of time, your risks are minimal. Even if you're on the Pill for more than ten years, your risk of breast cancer may increase, but that doesn't necessarily mean you'll get it. The birth control pills on the market today contain a lower dose of hormones than they did previously, so Pill users of today face a somewhat lower risk of breast cancer than Pill users of decades ago. Also, girls who start their periods when they're really young and stop them when they're really old are more at risk of breast cancer. Many factors come into play when talking about breast cancer. So it may be a combination of genetics, taking the Pill, and starting your period when you were very young that causes breast cancer. And who knows, if you hadn't taken the Pill, you may still have gotten breast cancer. The best we can say right now about a link between birth control pills and breast cancer is . . . maybe.

Kicking the Habit

Nobody wakes up one morning and suddenly decides to be a smoker. Smoking is a habit picked up from others who smoke. It's a social disease. Individuals do it in imitation of somebody they respect who smokes, like parents or teachers, or they do it because their high-school or college friends smoke and they want to fit in.

But once you put a cigarette in your mouth, you are exposed (not to mention that you are exposing everyone around you, as well) to the effects of nicotine, which is one of the mostly highly addictive drugs available today. And the more you smoke, the greater is your urge to smoke, and the more addicted you become.

The smoking habit will wreak havoc throughout the decades of your life because once you start to smoke, its deleterious effects spiral out of control, much like credit card debt. Smoking is associated not only with all kinds of cancer, from oral cancer to cervical cancer, but also with heart disease, which is the leading cause of death in the United States today for both men and women. Since smoking also affects the respiratory system, chronic smokers have a higher incidence of bronchitis (an inflammation of the lining of the tubes that connect the windpipe to the lungs) and emphysema (a chronic lung disease usually caused by exposure to toxic chemicals or tobacco smoke) than those who don't smoke. And smoking interferes with the immune system as well; that is, smokers are more prone to getting chronic diseases, flu, and viral illnesses than are nonsmokers. Then there are the secondary effects that smoking has on others. Pregnant women who smoke have smaller-sized babies and have higher rates of premature babies. And children who are exposed to secondhand smoke have higher levels of asthma.

If you are a smoker, there may be no better thing you can do for your health than to quit smoking, and the best time to quit is as a young adult. You may have started smoking in high school or college, but now you are on your own, away from the peer pressures of your schoolmates and the influence of your parents (who may be smokers themselves), and making a new life for yourself. This is the easiest time to kick the habit. Of course, quitting is easier said than done. As Mark Twain remarked: "Quitting smoking is easy. I've done it a thousand times." The reason it's so difficult to quit is that it's really a dual challenge, and you are unlikely to succeed in your quest unless you meet both challenges head-on.

The first challenge involves breaking the physical dependency that smoking causes. An absence of nicotine leads to withdrawal symptoms, including anxiety, nervousness, and an overwhelming desire for more nicotine. Very few people can go cold turkey and never pick up another cigarette again. Most people need to be gradually desensitized of their nicotine addiction. One way to do that is with Nicorette gum or the nicotine patch. These products allow you to alter, over a course of weeks, the amount of nicotine that you ingest, until your body gets used to having no nicotine at all. Acupuncture and hypnosis have also helped people reduce or eliminate the withdrawal symptoms—irritability, depression, and lack of energy—that come from kicking the nicotine habit.

The second challenge for the smoker seeking to quit involves breaking the mental habit that smoking reinforces. The best way to do that is through the same system that got you smoking in the first place, through a peer support system. Just as in overcoming any addiction, breaking the smoking habit requires a support group, which can consist of friends, family, and/or coworkers. But you have to have somebody who is willing to be there for you, to give you the support you need when you are most likely to want to pick up another cigarette.

Quitting should be celebrated at every little step of the way because you'll be seeing the benefits of your efforts in the minutes, days, weeks, months, and years after you quit. Twenty minutes after you smoke your last cigarette, your heart rate drops. Twelve hours later, the carbon monoxide level in your bloodstream returns to normal. Two to three weeks after quitting, your circulation improves, and your lungs begin to function normally. One year after you quit, the excess risk of coronary heart disease is half that of a smoker. In five years' time, your risk of stroke is reduced to that of a nonsmoker. In ten years' time, your risk of dying of lung cancer is about half that of a smoker. And in fifteen years, your risk of coronary heart disease is like that of someone who never smoked.

The long and short of it is, the sooner you quit, the quicker you'll regain your health.

Common Skin Conditions

Location, location, location is the mantra of real estate. When it comes to our greatest concern surrounding our appearance, the mantra is skin, skin, skin. Few people manage to sail through life without experiencing one sort of skin problem or another, acne being the most common. But millions of Americans suffer from a variety of more serious skin conditions.

Eczema

Other than acne, *eczema* may be the most common skin problem in the United States. Estimates of the number of people who have eczema range from 15 million to 30 million, a disparity that probably results from the fact that eczema can vary from mild—resulting in dry, hot, and itching skin—to severe—resulting in raw, blistered, and cracked skin.

Because there are multiple types of eczema, there are multiple causes.

Why Quit?

It's the fourth leading cause of death in the United States, claiming the lives of more than 120,000 people a year. About 16 million Americans have chronic obstructive pulmonary disease (COPD), a chronic lung disease that involves two distinct diseases: chronic bronchitis and emphysema. In chronic bronchitis, the lining in your bronchial tubes or airways becomes inflamed and full of mucus, which makes it hard to breathe. In emphysema, your alveoli, or air sacs in the lungs, are irritated. This causes the alveoli to stiffen, which means they can't hold enough air, and that makes it hard for you to get oxygen into and carbon dioxide out of your blood. There is very little mystery about what causes COPD; tobacco smoke is responsible for 80 to 90 percent of COPD cases. There is no cure for it. Only by stopping smoking can someone with COPD stop, or at least slow, the damage to their lungs. If you don't smoke, don't start. If you do, stop right now.

The most common type is *atopic dermatitis,* a genetic condition usually associated with such allergies as asthma and hay fever. It usually appears at a very young age, even in babies, though it often improves considerably with age, and in some cases may disappear completely. *Contact dermatitis* is a type of eczema caused by contact with an irritant of some kind or an allergen. This usually develops when individuals reach their thirties or later and often continues through adulthood.

While eczema cannot be cured, it can be controlled, usually by avoiding the allergens or other substances that irritate the skin. To learn just which specific substance affects you is typically a lengthy process of elimination, which requires the help of a dermatologist. Those who suffer from eczema usually also avoid exposure to dust and sand, perfumes and other cosmetics, soaps and detergents, wool fibers, and cigarette smoke, all of which can exacerbate their condition.

Treatment of eczema aims to stop flare-ups and heal the skin. Mild symptoms are usually treated with over-the-counter moisturizing creams and ointments, and over-the-counter antihistamines are used to control the itching. The skin infections caused by eczema are treated with antibiotics. More severe cases of eczema require more powerful medications that only a doctor can prescribe.

Psoriasis

Psoriasis is an inflammatory skin condition characterized by patches of thick, red skin covered with silvery scales. These occur primarily on the scalp, lower back, elbows, knees, and legs, and usually appear in people between the ages of fifteen and thirty-five. Psoriasis affects more than 4 million people. It's basically an acceleration of the normal cycle of skin generation, in which cells grow, die, and flake off; instead of this cycle's happening over a period of weeks, it occurs over a matter of days. In psoriasis, a natural layer of dead skin never gets a chance to form.

Psoriasis can be uncomfortable, sometimes painful, and often emotionally distressing. It's a chronic disease that affects men and women equally, with lesions often flaring up for weeks and months, followed by periods of remission in which the lesions subside or disappear entirely before coming back again. In some cases psoriasis lesions have been associated with symptoms of arthritis.

Though scientists do not fully understand what causes psoriasis, they now believe that it is an immune-system-mediated condition. It appears that the immune system's *T cells*—white blood cells that spring into action to fight off viruses and bacteria—suddenly respond to an individual's own skin cells as if they were foreign invaders. Just why the T cells misfire in this manner and set off a proliferation of new skin is not known, but clearly both environmental and genetic factors are involved. Stress, an injury to the skin, strep throat, excessive sun exposure, and certain medications for high blood pressure or bipolar disorder, for example, may trigger the condition, particularly in people with a hereditary predisposition for psoriasis. About one-third of the people who develop this skin condition have at least one family member with it, too.

There is no cure for psoriasis, and treatment can be incredibly challenging given its cycles of exacerbation and remission. Popular treatments include such topical ointments as steroids, vitamin D, cold tar, moisturizers, and retinoids that are used to treat acne, as well as natural or artificial ultraviolet light.

Vitiligo

In *vitiligo,* another skin condition, the skin loses its melanin, the pigment that colors the skin—and protects it from damage from ultraviolet light—and colors your hair and eyes as well. As the colorizing cells in your body die prematurely, you begin to develop the white patches of skin that are the hallmark of vitiligo. This condition usually first appears between the ages of twenty and thirty on sun-exposed areas of the skin. Some early signs of vitiligo include the premature whitening and graying of the hair, scalp, eyelashes, eyebrows, and beard. You may even lose the pigmentation of your eyes. Any part of your body may be affected; it can be limited to one area of the body or one side of the body, or it can be widespread. Most people with vitiligo are otherwise healthy. The condition tends to run in the family and may be more common in people with autoimmune diseases such as Addison's disease, vitamin B$_{12}$ deficiency, anemia, and hyperthyroidism.

Though there is no cure for vitiligo, there are treatments that can help restore some of the pigment of the skin. These include steroid creams and the use of ultraviolet light to darken the light patches of skin, as well as depigmentation, which involves fading the rest of your skin to match the color of the light patches. Tattooing is another possible solution, as are surgical skin grafts, which involve taking a piece of unaffected skin from one area and putting it in the affected area. People with vitiligo have to protect their skin, especially the fair patches, from the sun.

Rosacea

Rosacea is an inflammatory skin condition that can cause a redness of the face. You can mistake rosacea, especially if it's very small, with acne, but it isn't. It affects 14 million Americans. It often begins as a tendency to blush easily, and is caused by a dilation of the blood vessels close to the skin's surface. As the disease progresses, the small blood vessels on the nose and cheeks may swell and become visible in a kind of spiderweb pattern, and, eventually, if left untreated, the rosacea may turn into persistent inflammatory bumps or postules, which may need to be surgically removed.

The cause of rosacea is unknown. Some believe it is a chronic bacterial infection that's similar to *H. pylori,* the gastrointestinal bacteria that causes ulcers. Environmental factors may also be involved, though it's clear that extreme temperatures, sunlight, stress, hot baths, steroids, and spicy food can all aggravate rosacea. One thing is certain: it's not caused by alcohol.

Rosacea won't go away by itself and should be treated. The most effective treatment is a topical antibiotic that essentially prevents the bacteria from overgrowing. Sometimes oral antibiotics are needed when the lesions are severely inflamed. Once the rosacea is treated, the skin must be well protected. Use sunscreen, avoid skin irritants and facial products that are alcohol-based, and in the wintertime protect your face from the cold weather by using a face mask.

Autoimmune but (Thankfully) Not Automatic

Few young adults suffer serious health problems, though a continuation of bad habits—overeating, not getting enough exercise, and abusing drugs, including alcohol and cigarettes—in this decade pretty much guarantees trouble a decade or so down the road. The exception to this healthy young-adult rule occurs when you are born with a genetic autoimmune disease like lupus or sarcoidosis.

Lupus

Lupus is the great imitator. It can look like arthritis. It can look like mononucleosis. It can look like a whole raft of diseases. It is a disease with many faces, and not a single pleasant one among them. Lupus is a long-lasting, crippling disease in which the immune system, for unknown reasons, goes into overdrive and begins to attack the normal tissue of the body—liver, kidneys, and the like. Because the immune system is attacking itself and the rest of the body, it is called an *auto*immune disease.

To understand lupus you really have to understand a little bit about the immune system. Our immune system is designed to defend and protect the body against foreign intruders like bacteria and viruses. It's like our internal police system. Now imagine this internal police system being corrupt and actually *attacking* the people whom it is supposed to serve. So, like a corrupt police system, lupus attacks both the good and the bad because it doesn't know how to differentiate one from the other. It carries out those attacks by creating antibodies that disperse and travel through the blood and interact with normal body tissues, where it causes inflammation.

Lupus is ten to fifteen times more common in women than in men, and it usually begins to appear during the childbearing years. But unless the lupus is so severe that it has already damaged the mother's vital organs such as her kidney, or liver, most women, under adequate obstetrical care, can bear children without problems. People of all races can get lupus, though the incidence among African American women is three times higher than among Caucasian women. Asian, Hispanic, and Native American women also experience a higher-than-average rate of lupus. There is also a very rare type of lupus called *neonatal lupus,* and sometimes people develop lupus after drugs damage their immune system; that's called drug-induced lupus. And there's a lupus variety that mainly attacks the skin.

Lupus has many symptoms, but most people with lupus don't necessarily experience them all. Some of the symptoms include achy and swelling joints, persistent low-grade fever, fatigue, skin rashes (typically what they call the butterfly rash on the face), chest pain while breathing deeply, anemia, protein in the urine, hair loss, sensitivity to light, blood-clotting problems, blue or pale fingers especially in the cold weather, seizures, and ulcers in the mouth and nose that last longer than two weeks.

Certain things can trigger a lupus attack: ultraviolet light or sun poisoning, certain prescription drugs, infection, certain antibiotics, hormones, and, yes, even stress. There are also fears that breast implants, especially silicon breast implants, and the use of aspartame, the artificial sweetener, may also be linked to lupus, but no evidence of any such links has been found to date.

Lupus is difficult to diagnose because its symptoms can mimic so many other types of diseases. It also doesn't develop rapidly, and in its early phases it displays no symptoms. Since there is no single test that can measure with any degree of accuracy whether or not lupus is the cause of a person's symptoms, most physicians must diagnose lupus on the basis of medical history, symptoms, and laboratory analysis. But sometimes it can take up to ten years before enough symptoms accumulate that a doctor can make a definitive diagnosis of lupus.

What can patients with lupus do to improve their immune system? One is follow a healthy diet. There is no specific lupus diet, but patients with lupus should adhere to a diet that is rich in vegetables, low in refined sugars, low in fat, and high in fiber. Multivitamins are okay, but people with lupus should not take vitamins excessively. Good exercise, like walking, swimming, and bicycling, especially when lupus symptoms are not present, is encouraged. But when the symptoms of fatigue and tiredness appear in lupus patients, they should listen to their body and take a nap. The body is telling them that it's tired and needs to rest. One of the natural ways that bodies heal is through sleep. If you have lupus, it is particularly important to get a full eight hours of sleep. And if you're taking medication, always take it as recommended. Do not think that because you feel well you should stop your medication. Sometimes lupus goes into remission. If it does, you should continue to monitor your symptoms and see your doctor on a regular basis.

Lupus is not contagious and certainly cannot be transmitted sexually. Though not usually fatal, an individual can die from the complications of lupus, usually from infection because there's no way of fighting off disease, or from kidney failure. But today, with early treatment, 80 percent of people with lupus can expect to live a normal life span. If you have a mild case of lupus, with little more than the symptoms of inflammation and joint pain, a doctor will usually recommend a nonsteroidal inflammatory medicine, like naproxen (Aleve, for example) or ibuprofen. Those with a more severe case of lupus will need steroidal medicines like corticosteroids to slow down their hyperactive immune system, but taking steroids can increase appetite and cause weight gain. Steroids also cause a loss of bone mass, so there's a concern with regard to early development of osteoporosis and early need of hip replacement, for example. A life with lupus will not necessarily be trouble-free, but chances are you'll be around just as long as those lucky friends of yours who don't have lupus.

Sarcoidosis

All autoimmune diseases have similar underlying causes and conditions, and all are treated in a similar fashion. What distinguishes *sarcoidosis* from the other autoimmune diseases is the development of granulomas, or well-circumscribed, enlarged tissues, almost like big pimples, found on the skin, in the lungs, on the spleen, on the liver, on the reproductive organs—basically on any organ of the body.

Many people present little more than a mild form of sarcoidosis, in which the granulomas stop growing or shrink, and may disappear entirely in a few years. In others the inflammation that causes the granulomas remains but doesn't worsen. And in some, the sacoidosis becomes steadily worse over the years and can cause permanent organ damage.

Though the root cause of sarcoidosis is not well understood, the immune system most certainly plays a role, as granulomas are primarily made up of cells from the immune system. Some recent research indicates that the bacteria in granulomas may be the cause of sarcoidosis. Consequently, antibiotics may be an effective treatment for some people. In other patients, corticosteroids seem to slow or reverse the course of the disease, but then other patients do not respond at all to steroid therapy. Sarcoidosis lesions on the skin are sometimes treated with topical antibiotic ointments in order to eradicate secondary infections that may develop. Pain relievers are prescribed for patients who have arthritic symptoms relating to sarcoidosis.

Because these lesions tend to grow over time, those affected by the disease may show no symptoms, or, if the lesions get large enough, they may interfere with the normal functioning of the organ on which they are located. In the chest area, for instance, they can cause disturbed heart rhythms. Sarcoidosis is commonly found in the lungs, where it produces symptoms such as wheezing, shortness of breath, dry cough, or breathing pains. Often the disease is found by accident on an X-ray, especially on a chest X-ray when somebody goes in for a routine physical. Other people have skin sarcoidosis, big bumps on the face or discolored skin.

Early diagnosis is the key to the treatment of sarcoidosis. To halt its

WHAT IS GOING ON HERE?

One of the puzzling things about sarcoidosis, other than its cause, is just who gets it. In the United States, African Americans are ten to seventeen times more likely to get it than whites. Yet in Europe, it's mostly whites who are affected. How can this be? Here are the numbers of people who get the disease per one hundred thousand in the following countries:

Poland: 3
France: 10
Sweden: 64
Irish women living in London: 200

Now here's the real puzzler. Let's say a person from Poland, where there is a low incidence of sarcoidosis, leaves for an area with a high prevalence of the disease, like Sweden. That person will now face the same risk of the disease as anyone in Sweden! Figure it out, and a Nobel Prize may be yours.

progress, doctors recommend a healthy lifestyle of balanced nutrition, vitamin supplements, minimal exposure to the sun, and low levels of stress. The good news is that, more than half the time, sacoidosis cures itself within a year or two.

The Long Winding Road (Gastrointestinal Disorders)

The gastrointestinal (GI) tract is an organ that starts with our lips and ends at our anus. The long tract of tissue in between consists of the mouth, esophagus, stomach, small intestine, large intestine, rectum, and anus. Basically, that long winding road, which is known as the GI tract for short, is responsible for digesting and processing everything that we eat and converting it into the energy that our bodies need to function. But as with any plumbing system, the GI tract is prone to leaks, backups, and other disturbances.

GERD

As we age, one of the most common disturbances of the GI tract occurs at the bottom of the esophagus, the tube that connects the mouth to the stomach, where a valve, or ring of muscle called a sphincter, normally keeps contents of the stomach—the food, acid, and bile—in the stomach where it belongs and out of the esophagus and away from our breathing tube. When this lower esophageal sphincter does not close properly, however, the contents of the stomach back up, or reflux, into the esophagus. When acid from the stomach comes into contact with the lining of the esophagus, a burning sensation, which is called heartburn, occurs in the chest or throat. When this fluid is tasted in the back of the mouth, it is called acid indigestion. Occasional heartburn is common. But if it occurs more than twice a week, the acidity of the stomach can damage the esophagus and may be a sign of gastroesophageal reflux disease, or GERD, which can lead to more serious health problems like esophageal cancer.

No one knows exactly why people get GERD, but doctors are aware of several factors that may contribute to the disease. Certain anatomical deformities of the esophagus or the stomach may lead the sphincter to malfunction and allow the contents of the stomach to migrate easily into the esophagus. One condition that would allow this return of acid would be a *hiatal hernia,* which occurs when the upper part of the stomach protrudes above the diaphragm (the muscle that separates the chest from the abdomen). But most of the time the factors that are associated with this reflux of acid are usually of our own making. Here we're talking about using alcohol, being overweight, smoking, and yes, being pregnant. There are also many foods that increase the amount of acid we have in our stomach. Citrus fruits, chocolate, coffee, fried foods, garlic and onions, as well as tomato-based products like spaghetti sauce and pizza, can all make a bad situation worse.

Treating GERD requires some lifestyle changes. If you smoke, stop. If you drink excessive amounts of alcohol, tone it down. If you are overweight, lose some pounds. It's also a good idea to pace your meals, and you shouldn't lie down for three hours after eating a meal. When you do go to bed or lie down, get some help from gravity by raising your head about eight inches, or two pillows' worth, from a horizontal position.

Unless you are a hermit or live without a TV, you can't help but be aware of all the possible medications you can take to alleviate the problem. For mild cases, there are a host of over-the-counter antacids, such as Rolaids, Tums, Alka-Seltzer, Maalox, and Pepto-Bismol. Most of these antacids neutralize the acidity in your stomach with a combination of three basic salts—magnesium, calcium, and aluminum—and hydroxide or bicarbonate ions. Also available are what are called the H2 blockers, such as Tagamet, Pepcid, or Zantac, all of which impede acid production. And now there is yet another generation of medications called proton pump inhibitors, including Prilosec, Prevacid, or Nexium. These medications are even more effective than the H2 blockers in preventing the formation of acid in the stomach. Not only can they act quickly and dramatically improve the symptoms, they can actually begin to heal any chronic inflammation that might have already developed in the lower esophagus.

If the symptoms persist, additional diagnostic tests may be needed to determine the root cause of your particular problem. Typical diagnostic tests to rule out problems of the GI tract include a barium X-ray, in which you drink a liquid that allows various features of the esophagus to appear in an X-ray; and an upper endoscopy, in which a small tube is threaded down your throat into your esophagus and stomach to allow the doctor to see the inner lining of your upper digestive system. In very rare cases—if the discomfort is chronic and debilitating—surgery may be necessary to repair the stomach. This is now usually done with minimally invasive surgery that allows the patients to return home relatively quickly.

Diarrhea

Another common problem with the digestive system is diarrhea. Everybody has experienced those loose, watery stools, that send you scurrying to the bathroom several times a day and that last a day or so before going away. It might seem like just a temporary inconvenience, but the real problem with diarrhea is that your body loses a lot of fluid, which contains electrolytes, those essential salts that your cells use to carry out nerve and muscle functions. So, ultimately, the problem with diarrhea is one of dehydration, particularly for older folks and young children. The major signs of dehydration are poor urine function, disorientation, heart palpitations, and generalized fatigue.

There are many reasons for diarrhea. Water or food contaminated with common bacteria, such as salmonella and *E. coli,* can cause diarrhea. So can many viruses, like the rotavirus, the Norwalk virus, and the hepatitis virus. Some people have diarrhea due to food allergies that prevent them from digesting certain foods such as lactose, the sugar found in milk. Various parasites can cause diarrhea, too, as can some antibiotics and blood pressure medications. Colitis and Crohn's disease can cause diarrhea, too.

If you have significant fever, 102°F or greater, associated with your diarrhea, or if there is blood in your stool, you should seek immediate medical attention, as these could be signs of a major infection. You should also consult a doctor if you have had diarrhea for more than three days, or if you are experiencing significant pain or discomfort, especially in the rectal area. A doctor will conduct a physical exam, do a blood test, and take a stool culture in an attempt to find the source of the diarrhea. If no cause is readily apparent, the doctor may recommend a diagnostic test such as a colonoscopy, in which a tube with a camera is inserted into the rectum for a detailed examination of the large intestine.

Treating diarrhea means first treating the dehydration. You have to drink lots of fluids. Water is best to replace those lost electrolytes, as coffee, tea, and other caffeinated beverages can increase dehydration, and fruit juices and sodas can actually make diarrhea worse. If the diarrhea is

What does a sixteenth-century emperor of Mexico have to do with it?

It's known by a variety of colorful names—Ghandi's revenge, gyppy tummy, Delhi belly, Rangoon runs, Tokyo trots, gringo gallop, Aztec two-step, and Montezuma's revenge—all of which reflect the embarrassment felt by the sufferer traveling in a foreign land. This bacteriological illness, more formally known as "traveler's diarrhea," is usually caused by drinking contaminated water or eating spicy food to which one is not accustomed.

To prevent traveler's diarrhea, don't drink the tap water; don't even brush your teeth with it. Drink and use bottled water only. Don't drink unpasteurized milk or other diary products, stay away from ice cream, and avoid having ice in your drinks. Do not eat any rare or raw meat or fish. Do not eat shellfish, even if it's hot. And avoid all raw fruits and vegetables.

Remember always to bring along some antidiarrheal medicine like Imodium AD if you must live on the wild side.

due to a virus, it will eventually go away. If the diarrhea is due to a bacterial infection, the doctor will prescribe a course of antibiotics.

To recover from a bout of diarrhea, you will also need to adjust your diet temporarily. It's best to start with nothing more than clear liquids. Avoid milk products, high-fiber products, and very sugary products. As the symptoms improve, moderate your diet over several days from bland soft foods to simply bland foods before returning to regular food.

In the end, it's important to remember that diarrhea is a common problem that's usually resolved on its own.

Crohn's Disease

Severe diarrhea may be a sign of inflammatory bowel disease (IBD), which can lead to life-threatening complications. Both Crohn's disease and ulcerative colitis are IBDs that can cause an inflammation of the lining of the digestive tract, creating severe abdominal pain and bouts of watery or bloody diarrhea. But while ulcerative colitis affects only the innermost lining of the large intestine and rectum, Crohn's disease can occur anywhere in the colon and does so by spreading deeply into the affected tissue.

Crohn's disease affects anywhere from a half million to a million Americans and has no known medical cure. This autoimmune bowel disease causes the cells of the infected area of the intestines to secrete large amounts of water and salt, which the colon cannot absorb; the water and salt build up in the intestines, eventually causing diarrhea, debilitating abdominal cramps, and dehydration. The blood in the stool can lead to severe anemia, and, of course, this ultimately results in a lack of appetite and tremendous weight loss. Then fatigue sets in from the lack of nutrients and the poor absorption of fluids and electrolytes.

Crohn's disease mostly strikes people in their twenties, with diagnosis usually occurring between the ages of fifteen and thirty-five. It's more prevalent in whites than in blacks, and if you're of Jewish or European descent, you are four to five times more likely to develop the disease. Latinos don't develop Crohn's, however. There appears to be a genetic aspect to Crohn's disease: about 20 percent of people diagnosed with Crohn's disease have a parent, sibling, or child who has the disease. Environmental factors, a high-fat diet, refined foods, and refined carbohydrates may also play a role.

There is also some evidence to suggest that a virus or bacteria may cause Crohn's disease. Almost like an allergic reaction, the invasive microorganism not only activates the immune system but causes it to go into overdrive, inflaming the digestive system in the process. Both colonoscopies and CAT scans can reveal the inflammation associated with Crohn's disease very clearly.

If the dehydration and anemia that accompany the disease are not treated, Crohn's disease can be life-threatening. Obstructions are another complication of Crohn's disease; the mucosa of the bowel can become so inflamed that it almost completely obstructs the flow of food in the intestines. The inflammation can also lead to open sores or ulcers, which, if they extend completely through the intestinal wall, may create fistulas or abnormal connections between different parts of your intestines, sometimes causing a drainage of bowel contents through your skin. Because Crohn's affects the whole body, some people will develop arthritis, kidney stones or gallstones, early osteoporosis, and, of course, colon cancer.

The goal of treating Crohn's disease is to reduce the inflammation. Steroids and other drugs are usu-

Irritable Bowels

IBS, or irritable bowel syndrome, is also known as spastic colon, spastic colitis, nervous stomach, or irritable colon. This disorder is thought to affect 10 to 15 percent of the population, and, for reasons unknown, women suffer from IBS twice as often as men. Characterized by lower abdominal pain, diarrhea, constipation, bloating, gas, nausea, and back pain, IBS can be a mild inconvenience to some, while an agonizing experience for others. Since there are many other conditions that can produce similar bowel symptoms, such as bowel cancer, endometriosis, fibromyalgia, intestinal parasites, Crohn's disease, and ulcerative colitis, only a doctor, preferably a board-certified gastroenterologist, can rule out these alternatives and properly diagnose a case of IBS. While there is no cure for this disorder, most sufferers, with the help of their doctor, can find something, either dietary, medicinal, or both, to manage the problem.

ally prescribed to reduce this inflammation, while other medications are given to suppress the immune system's overenergetic response. Antibiotics are prescribed to heal the fistulas, pain relievers to relieve the debilitating pain, and vitamin injections to prevent anemia.

While there is no evidence that what you eat actually causes the disease, certain foods and beverages can aggravate the symptoms. You want to limit dairy products, eat low-fat foods in small meals, and drink plenty of liquids. It's important to consult a dietitian. Even though it was long thought that stress was strongly linked to Crohn's disease, we know now that there is no relation between the two, though stress can certainly exacerbate the symptoms. Consequently, exercise, yoga, relaxation techniques, and hypnosis can help reduce the stress and better manage the disease and its symptoms.

Constipation

Einstein would never admit it, but there is nothing more relative in this world than people's bathroom habits. Many people are confused about what "normal bowel habits" really mean. The answer is: Anything from three times a day to three times a week. Admittedly, that's a *wide* range, and it suggests that what most people consider to be constipation—which is the infrequent evacuation of dry hardened feces from the bowels— probably isn't. And given the fact that Americans spend three-quarters of a billion dollars on laxatives each year, it also means that people are probably overusing and abusing laxatives.

Constipation is the most common gastrointestinal complaint in America, and it results in about 2 million visits to the doctor each year. Some 80 percent of the population has suffered from constipation at some point in life, and women report more constipation than do men.

Our bowel movements are affected by both diet and habit, and two factors in particular have a tremendous influence on what we do and don't do when it comes to bowel movements. One is the more fiber you eat, the

The Poop on Fiber

Many vegetables, fruits, and grains are high in fiber, which helps form soft bulky stool and prevent constipation.

Raw Vegetables	Fruits	Other Foods
Acorn squash	Apples	Whole-grain cereals
Broccoli	Peaches	Whole-wheat bread
Brussels sprouts	Raspberries	Seven-grain bread
Cabbage	Tangerines	Lima beans
Carrots		Kidney beans
Cauliflower		Black-eyed peas
Zucchini		

more regular you are. The typical American diet includes about 12 to 15 grams of fiber a day, which is nowhere near the recommended amout of 25 to 30 grams of fiber a day. The same goes for water; we just don't drink enough liquid to maintain proper bowel function. Are you drinking at least eight to ten cups of fluid a day? You should be.

Another factor contributing to constipation is, again, a lack of exercise. The older we get, the less mobile we are; our intestines need a certain amount of activity to move all the roughage necessary to maintain a normal bowel function. Travel, pregnancy, and stress may also aggravate constipation. Some medical diseases are associated with increased constipation, including lupus, thyroid disease, multiple sclerosis, Parkinson's disease, and stroke. Likewise, some medications have been linked to constipation, especially painkillers, narcotics, antidepressants, tranquilizers, and blood pressure medicines.

Brief periods of constipation are normal. But if you experience a dramatic shift in bowel habits, in either frequency or size, if you are constipated for more than three weeks, or if there is blood in your stool, then by all means see a doctor right away. The doctor will do a physical examination, check for anatomical problems, like a narrowing of the intestinal tract, and look for polyps or tumors or diverticular disease, in which small pouches bulge out through weak spots in the colon.

Whatever you do, don't become a laxative addict. Some people become so dependant on laxatives that they can't have a bowel movement without them. The key to preventing and dealing with constipation is to develop regular bowel habits, by increasing the fiber in your diet, pacing your intake of food, and drinking lots of liquids. And don't forget to shake your booty every now and then.

Three Decades Down, the Number Left Is up to You

By the end of the decade of the twenties, the aging process has begun. Yes, it has, though not noticeably so. Muscle bulk and strength start to decline. The brain starts to age as well. The liver may have taken a hit trying to detoxify the drugs and alcohol in your system. The senses remain sharp, although hearing may be stressed from exposure to high-decibel noises from concerts and personal music players. The skin, while no longer as fresh as a baby's bottom, should not show any age deterioration at this point in life, unless it has been excessively exposed to the sun. (See "Skin Health and Cancer," page 139.)

It's difficult to think about health issues when you're firing on all cylinders, as you are in your twenties. But you're not invincible. What you do, or don't do, now will have a profound effect ten to twenty years down the road. Just remember that the key to a healthy life is really quite simple: Eat well, though not a lot; exercise regularly, particularly if you have a sedentary job; and stay away from drugs, including cigarettes and alcohol. Contrary to what you might think, they are not doing you any favors.

Test Checklist for this Decade

	Check BMI
	STDs/HIV tests
	Tetanus booster
	Gynecological exam (yearly)
	Dental cleaning (yearly)
	Cholesterol test (every five years, for men, if at risk)
	Check blood pressure (every two years)
	Breast self-examination (monthly)
	Skin check (every three months)
	Mental health screening (for depression, if needed)

Living Responsibly

4

It's a time of increased responsibility. Work pressures increase, as do family commitments—bringing up a child and owning a home, perhaps. And for the first time health issues start showing up on your radar. Good thing, too. When it comes to your health, these are often called the "make-or-break years."

Mentor

Check BM

STDs/HIV

Tetanus

Gyneco

Dental

Chole

Blood

Brea

Skin

Bas

Me

(fo

The life path starts diverging radically in the course of this decade. Some people have had children by now; others are just now starting to think about having a family, and still others have decided not to have children at all. Whether you have children or not plays a large role in how you live your life and how it affects your health. People without children are more likely to smoke and abuse alcohol and other drugs. Those who have children probably feel the impact of having a family on their work, their social life, and their relationship with their partner.

What it comes down to is a matter of time: what you choose to do with it, and whether or not health is on your agenda. My advice? If your health wasn't high on your priority list before, it had better be now. Balancing work and family can be time-consuming enough without having to find some time in your busy day to exercise for instance. That said, some say that these are the make-or-break years for long-term health. And in some ways that's true. For example, if you give up smoking by age thirty-five, your life expectancy will be pretty much the same as that of a person who never smoked. It's a presidential pardon of sorts. If you need it, take advantage of it now. But remember, when it comes to your health, it's never too late to make improvements. Any improvement you make at any time of your life will benefit your health immensely.

Nutrition

I think Americans generally pay more attention to the gasoline they put in their cars than to the food they put in their mouths. We are a society of excess, and one of our more impressive excesses is the way in which we eat and what we choose to put in our mouths. We are the leading country in the world in almost everything, yet our mortality rates, our cancer rates, and our neonatal death rates don't rank among the best in the world. We lead in research, we lead in academic training, we lead in freedom of information, yet we don't lead in taking care of our health. We have all the knowledge in the world about everything in life, but that has made no impact on our health. Why? I think nutrition is part of the reason, and I think I know why.

No one is ever taught about nutrition. We certainly don't teach the subject in grammar school, and it's rarely taught in high school. Some colleges may offer it as an elective. But our parents certainly don't talk to us about carbohydrates and proteins the way they do about the birds and the bees. If you combine this lack of knowledge with our appetite for diversity, taste, and presentation, what you have is a lot of people who know nothing about the food on their plate.

It's never too late to learn about nutrition. The fundamental issue with nutrition is learning how to balance your caloric intake with the number of calories you burn. Everything we eat has a caloric value. If you take in more nutrients that contain a lot of calories and you don't burn them up, the excess caloric energy is going to be stored as fat, and you're going to gain weight. That weight and that fat will then interfere with all the normal functions of your body. On the other hand, if you consume too few calories, say fewer than twelve hundred calories a day, then your body doesn't have sufficient energy to maintain adequate functioning. The caloric intake for a normal adult should range between fifteen hundred and two thousand calories a day.

The body requires certain nutrients in order to work properly. Nutrients are the chemicals our body gets from food. These nutrients are used to build muscles, improve cell-to-cell transmission, and manufacture hormones. In describing nutrients, the word "essential" means that the body must consume them; it cannot produce them on its own. The nutrients we need include:

- Essential amino acids. The body requires amino acids to produce new body proteins and replace damaged proteins to build and maintain the body.
- Vitamins and minerals. These are recognized as essential nutrients that are specifically linked to the functionality of cells. If we're deficient in vitamins and minerals, we develop a weak immune system, cell metabolism disorders, premature aging, scurvy, goiters, and bone loss.
- Fatty acids. Also essential, fatty acids are crucial for maintaining the body's normal health. They are responsible for the normal formation of hormones and creation of some of the biological pathways responsible for dealing with inflammation and cell repair.
- Sugars. They are essential because they provide the fuel our cells need to function adequately, which allows the other nutrients to be utilized properly. If cells don't have the sugar molecule necessary to generate the energy required for repairing, functioning, transmitting, and utilizing nutrients, then cellular damage and disease will result.

Each nutrient carries out one or more unique tasks your body needs to function. And because you need many nutrients to stay healthy—protein, fat, carbohydrates, vitamins, minerals—you have to eat a wide variety of foods to get them all. It's when we don't recognize the necessity of all those elements that we begin getting into trouble. It's like filling your gas tank with gasoline and forgetting to change the oil every thirty-five hundred miles, or forgetting to put water in the radiator. The car needs the gasoline, the oil and the water, all in the proper proportions, in order to function properly. The same is true of the human body. The problem, as I've mentioned before, is that about one-third of all American meals are prepared foods. And the problem with prepared foods is that their contents are not nutritionally balanced.

Our lack of knowledge of nutrition, combined with our obsession with processed foods, is really damaging our health. So we have to get back to fundamentals, a good example of which is the diet of people who live in the Mediterranean. Their diet is well balanced with vegetables and fruit, fish and lean meat, and the good unsaturated fats like olive oil. Today, many people think that if they stick to low-fat or nonfat foods, they won't gain weight. That's a myth, because gaining weight has to do with calorie intake. If you take a salad and you add cheese and eggs and everything else in the book, even if you select low-fat ingredients, you're still consuming a tremendous load of calories. And size matters, too; the size of your portions does make a difference in terms of the total amount of calories consumed. It's just a plain mathematical calculation.

There are no magical foods that are going to help you burn calories or increase your cell metabolism either. There is no such a thing as a food that is more active in the body than others. People think that eating a grapefruit each day or having cabbage soup for lunch is going to burn off their fat. But that's a myth. There is only one way to burn off those extra calories: exercise, any exercise at all.

How to Eat

It's not just *what* or *how much* we are eating that's the problem these days, it's the *way* most of us eat. Many people skip breakfast, gulp down a quick lunch at noon, and then consume a large meal at seven o'clock at night. Trouble is, they don't need all that fuel at night. They need a little bit throughout the day when they are active—either moving, thinking, or both. So what happens in the middle of the day if this is the way we eat? Without a supply of energy, our metabolism gets altered. Our blood sugar level is erratic. Our hormones go haywire trying to figure out where to obtain the fuel we need. People are always telling me, "I don't eat, so how come I'm not losing weight?" That's the answer. Their metabolism is out of whack, and they need to get it back in order.

Ideally, for optimal energy consumption and metabolism, you should eat small meals every three hours. So, for instance, if you have breakfast at seven o'clock in the morning, then you would have a snack at ten, lunch at one, a snack at four, and dinner at about seven o'clock at night. And, of course, you need to drink a lot of water in between because water is necessary for cellular metabolism. If you look at how the fuel is being burned during the day in this scenario, your metabolism is in continuous motion, and therefore your energy level stays up. You're burning very efficiently all the food you consume during the day.

Supplements

If you eat a balanced diet with fruits, vegetables, grains, fish, and all the rest, you don't need to take supplements. But how many of us really eat such a balanced diet? And even if we do, because we are all predisposed for certain diseases and the aging processes, being proactive and adding certain supplements to our diet may be a good idea. But before popping supplements like candies from a bag of M&M's, check with your doctor

 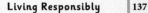

about what's best for you. Some supplements can be toxic. Others may cause allergies or cross reactions with medications you may be taking. But there is no doubt that certain supplements can have specific health benefits and can lower the cost of health care at the same time.

I am particularly bullish on five supplements that have been well studied and are proven to support optimal health. I love the omega-3 fatty acids. They are an important contributor to the improvement of human health. Some studies have shown that omega 3s are good for the prevention of heart disease, as well as for depression, rheumatoid arthritis, and asthma. You can get omega 3s by eating leafy greens and fish or by taking a fish oil tablet. Omega 3s assist with fat metabolism and help maintain a balance of good and bad cholesterol.

Calcium is another very good supplement, specifically calcium with vitamin D. Calcium intake is an important factor in bone health and may play a role in the prevention of colon cancer, though it doesn't appear to be the silver bullet that everyone hoped it would be. Research has shown that calcium supplements can significantly lower the occurrence of hip fractures among those aged sixty-five and older.

Folic acid and folate are forms of a water-soluble vitamin B that occur naturally in leafy vegetables such as spinach and turnip greens, dry beans and peas, fortified cereal products, and some other fruits and vegetables. Folic acid supplements have been a lifesaver in the prevention of neural tube defects in children. They are also very beneficial for cell function and the prevention of heart disease.

I also like glucosamine. It has good anti-inflammatory effects, especially for individuals with arthritis. It doesn't prevent arthritis, and it doesn't repair or rejuvenate cartilage, but I think it's a very good supplement because it helps promote joint function and relieves the symptoms of inflammation and pain.

Other supplements that are thought to make a positive contribution to health include saw palmetto, the fruit of the fan palm, for men. Native Americans consumed it as food and used it to treat urinary and genital problems. Some research has shown that it could be effective for the treatment of an enlarged prostate in men. It increases urinary flow and has no known safety hazards.

Skin Health and Cancer

You would never think so looking at it, but the skin is an organ just like the heart or the liver. In fact, it happens to be the largest organ in the body. The skin, as the border between the self and the outside world, is also the organ that defines us. It protects our internal organs from environmental threats. And for many people, the skin's appearance, the presence or lack of wrinkles, for instance, is what defines aging, more so than the condi-

THE SKINNY ON SKIN

Number of days it takes for the skin to renew itself: 28

Thickness of human skin in inches: 0.06 to 0.16

Average weight of adult male skin in pounds: 7

Surface area of adult male skin in square feet: 22

Millions of skin cells in average adult: 300

Number of hairs on a square half inch of skin: 10

Number of sweat glands in a square half inch of skin: 100

Number of feet of blood vessels in a square half inch of skin: 3.2

Number of days it takes for the skin to replace itself: 52 to 75

tion of their vital internal organs. Our skin is very important to us, but skin health is not something to which we give much (or any) thought.

As that part of our body that is the most exposed to the environment, the skin's greatest threat is the sun's rays, and overexposure to these rays appears to be the most important factor in the development of skin cancer, which is on the rise worldwide. One out of every five Americans will develop skin cancer, and nearly ten thousand will die from it each year. Skin cancer was long considered a problem only for people over fifty, but

Sunny Myths

Sunscreen protects you against all ultraviolet rays from the sun.

FALSE. It protects you from the sun's UVB rays, but no sunscreen product screens out all UVA rays, which are the cause of melanomas. So just because you put on sunscreen, you are not 100 percent protected.

You don't need to reapply sunscreen when you come out of the water if you use waterproof sunscreen lotions.

FALSE. There's no such a thing as a waterproof sunscreen. If you go into the water, you have to reapply these creams immediately because they get washed off.

Suntans are a sign of healthy skin.

FALSE. A tan is a sign of skin damage. The tanning occurs when the skin produces additional pigment (coloring) to protect itself against burns from the sun's ultraviolet rays.

in the last couple of decades, the rate of skin cancer for people in their forties and younger has multiplied explosively. You need to think about your skin before it's too late.

The sun produces two types of ultraviolet radiation. The ultraviolet A (UVA) rays, which penetrate deeper into the skin, are more responsible for melanoma, the most deadly type of skin cancer. The ultraviolet B (UVB) rays are responsible for sunburns and cause nonmelanomas, the squamous and basal cell skin cancers. Though melanomas account for only 4 percent of skin cancers, they are responsible for nearly 75 percent of all skin cancer deaths. Melanomas usually begin as flat, quarter-inch-sized, mottled, light brown to black blemishes with irregular borders. These blemishes can then turn red, blue, or white; crust on the surface; or bleed. Most frequently seen on the upper back, torso, lower legs, head, and neck, they can occur anywhere on the body.

While skin cancer is the most common type of cancer, and kills more young women than any other type of cancer, it is also the most preventable. The best defense against skin cancer is sun protection. Because the sun's ultraviolet rays can damage the cellular structure of the skin, the use of sun protection is important beginning at a young age and continuing throughout life. Whenever you are out in the sun, it's a good idea to use a sunscreen with a sun protection factor (SPF) of 15 or higher. Apply it fifteen to thirty minutes before going outdoors, and reapply it every two hours. If you can't avoid being out and about in the hours of peak sunlight—ten A.M. until four P.M.—seek the shade whenever possible and wear a hat, visor, sunglasses, and other protective clothing during prolonged periods of sun exposure.

Since skin cancer has a 95 percent cure rate when detected early, by your late thirties you should have

At Greater Risk

Anyone can get skin cancer, but you are at increased risk if you

- have a family history of skin cancer
- have many moles or large moles
- have naturally blond or red hair
- have blue or green eyes
- have had five or more sunburns
- have been overexposed to the sun early in life
- are Caucasian with fair skin

a skin physical every two years. This is particularly important if you are at greater risk for skin cancer (see "At Greater Risk," page 141). At a skin physical, a dermatologist will go over your entire body looking for atypical birthmarks, blemishes, and moles. This exam could save your life.

Skin cancers aside, chronic sun exposure also creates skin stains and premature wrinkling. Smoking, too, is bad for the skin. On the other hand, the aging of the skin can be slowed by a good diet. Certain foods, like salmon and the omega oils found in salmon, have been found to be extremely beneficial for skin health. On the other hand, while skin creams may reduce dryness, or improve excessive oiliness, they will not alter the overall health of the skin. Creams merely affect the superficial layer of the skin. Good skin health comes from within.

A Little Gland with a Big Job

For a small gland, the thyroid packs a punch. This small butterfly-shaped gland found in the neck just below the Adam's apple influences every organ, tissue, and cell in the body. In short, it controls our metabolism. The thyroid produces the hormones T3 and T4, which tell our body how to use energy. The "thermostat" that tells the thyroid how much hormone to produce is located in the base of our skull and is called the pituitary gland. When our thyroid hormone levels decrease or increase, the pituitary gland releases its own hormone, TSH, which, in turn, tells the thyroid to produce more or less thyroid hormone.

More than 20 million Americans suffer from either an overactive or an underactive thyroid gland. As many as half the cases of thyroid disease in the United States go undiagnosed. If left untreated, a diseased thyroid can elevate your cholesterol levels and cause infertility, muscle weakness, osteoporosis, and, in rare cases, coma or death.

Hyperthyroidism occurs when the thyroid produces too much hormone and our metabolism goes into overdrive. Some of the symptoms may include irritability, tremors, muscle weakness, weight loss, sleep disturbances, and an enlarged thyroid. One of the most common causes of hyperthyroidism is Grave's disease, or diffuse toxic goiter, an enlargement of the thyroid usually due to an autoimmune condition though sometimes unexplained. There are other causes of hyperthyroidism, such as a nodule within the thyroid gland that begins to release large quantities of hormones.

Hypothyroidism is the opposite of hyperthyroidism. In this condition, the thyroid gland makes too little thyroid hormone, and our metabolism slows down. Symptoms include fatigue, weight gain, a hoarse voice, an intolerance to cold, and menstrual irregularities. One of the most common reasons for hypothyroidism is an inflammation of the thyroid, which is called thyroiditis. This condition usually involves the immune system; antibodies are produced against the thyroid gland, which interfere with its normal function.

One of the key elements needed for a normal thyroid function is iodine. Too much or too little iodine can alter the hormone levels. Although this condition has been corrected in industrialized societies with the introduction of iodized salt, it is still very prevalent in many areas of the world.

The diagnosis of thyroid disease is relativity easy to make, usually by checking the levels of hormone such as TSH. If an enlarged thyroid gland is suspected, imaging tests such as ultrasound or MRI can confirm the diagnosis. If a tumor is suspected, a biopsy will be needed for confirmation; effective treatment is available, including surgery.

Hormone replacement therapy (HRT), usually a synthetic hormone called levothyroxine, is the key management tool for a hypoactive thyroid. In cases of hyperactive thyroid, reducing the amount of hormone regulates the thyroid gland. In such cases radioactive iodine, which disables the thyroid, is prescribed. Thyroid surgery is reserved for hyperactive areas of the thyroid, where a nodule is producing large quantities of hormone.

Though thyroid disease is a lifelong condition, when properly treated people can live healthy, normal lives. Both men and women should be screened for thyroid disease after the age of thirty-five.

Bladder Infections

Did you know that urine is normally sterile? When urine becomes contaminated, you have a bladder infection, otherwise known as a urinary tract infection, or UTI. These are very common in women due to the anatomy of the female pelvis. The female urethra is very short, compared to the male urethra, which is extended by the penis. Women tend to have more bladder infections in their thirties because many have had children by that age; vaginal deliveries can loosen their vaginal support and make them more prone to bladder infections. In men, an uncircumcised penis has been associated with an increase in bladder infections. But a bacterial infection of the prostate is the most common cause of bladder infections in men.

There are basically five reasons for bladder infections in women. First, soaps can cause an irritation and burning of the urethra, which is the outer opening of the tube that connects to the bladder. Second, it's quite common for women not to empty their bladder in a timely fashion. This occurs often with professional women who are constantly running around and never have time to go to the bathroom. Holding the urine in the bladder creates a potential for bacterial growth. Third, many people have anatomical abnormalities of the urinary system. Sometimes they have smaller, longer, or crooked urethra and bladders; any anatomical deformity that doesn't allow the urine to empty adequately can lead to bladder infections. Fourth, women suffering from constipation can experience bladder infections because hardened stool in the rectum can press against the bladder in such a way that it fails to empty adequately. And fifth, improper wiping can drag bacteria from the anal area to the urethra.

The symptoms of a bladder infection include burning, pain, frequent or urgent urination of a small amount at the time, fever, blood in the urine, and foul-smelling urine. If not treated promptly, the infection can travel through the bladder, through the ureters, and into the kidneys, where it can cause a kidney infection called a pyelonephritis, which should be taken seriously. Lower back pain, fever, and vomiting are signs of a kidney infection.

Doctors can diagnose bladder infections from the signs and symptoms. They can also do what is called a *clean catch*, in which they collect urine

Better Bladder Health

As always, prevention is the best medicine. Follow these four steps for victory over urinary tract infections.

1. Urinate frequently.

Help flush the bacteria, parasites, and other critters out of your system by going to the bathroom regularly—at least whenever you feel the urge—and drain your bladder completely each time. Remember to urinate after intercourse, too, as sexual activity can push foreign organisms into the uretha, the canal through which urine is discharged from the bladder.

2. Drink lots of fluids.

Water is excellent. Old remedies, like cranberry juice, will not cure bladder infections but may help prevent them. The acidity of the cranberry juice may prevent bacteria and other foreign organisms from sticking to the lining of the bladder and may also inhibit bacterial growth by acidifying urine.

3. Avoid UTI triggers.

Soaps and bath oils that irritate you. Tight underpants. Constipation.

4. Practice proper hygiene.

Wipe from front to back after a bowel movement; bacteria from the rectal area are the cause of many urinary tract infections.

with a tiny catheter tube inserted into the bladder through the urethra to see if it contains any bacteria. A urine analysis will also show the bacteria, and a blood test should show nitrites, which is a by-product of bacteria, if a bladder infection is present.

Bladder infections are treated with antibiotics. Usually a five- to seven-day course of antibiotics that's sensitive to the bacteria in your culture is sufficient to knock out the infection. Women who experience two or more episodes of urinary tract infections within a six-month period may need to be on a regular course of low-dose antibiotics. If you have recurrent infections, a doctor will have to check for anatomical deformities, which may require surgery.

Are You Collecting Stones?

The tables are turned when it comes to kidney stones. Men are more prone to kidney stones than women because they have a longer plumbing system—which consists of kidneys, ureter, bladder, and urethra—that permits the buildup of these stones.

Kidney stones are one of the most common and most painful disorders of the urinary tract, with more than a half million people going to emergency rooms for this problem every year. Kidney stones are formed from crystals that separate from the urine and build up on the inner surfaces of the kidney. Many times these crystals are very small and pass through the urethra painlessly. But sometimes they build up like tartar on your teeth, and once they get large enough, they can cause excruciating pain, bloody urine, nausea, vomiting, fevers, and the inability to urinate.

People prone to getting kidney stones have an imbalance of salts and minerals in their diet and, thus, in their urine. Different kinds of stones can form from the salts in the urine. Calcium stones, which are made of calcium (from dairy products and leafy green vegetables) and oxilate (from chocolate, tea, coffee, spinach, and strawberries), are the most common type of kidney stones. So one way to prevent them is to examine your diet; is there too much calcium in your diet? An excess of vitamin D could also be the reason. Certain diseases, such as an overactive parathyroid gland or sarcoidosis, can make extra calcium in your body. Other stones are made of uric acid, which is caused by eating a lot of meat. People who have gout or people who have received chemotherapy can develop uric acid stones. People with chronic kidney infections may have a buildup of ammonia in their system from the bacteria, and ammonia can build up and create a stone as well.

The average age of onset for kidney stones is during the thirties. It tends to run in families. Certain medications, like excessive use of calcium-based antacids, thyroid medication, and water pills increase the risk for kidney stones. Not surprisingly, anatomical deformities, like being born with only one kidney rather than two, can also affect the formation of kidney stones. A high-protein, low-fiber diet can contribute to stone formation, as can dehydration, lack of exercise, and poor mobility, which just allows things to build up in your system.

A doctor who suspects kidney stones from the symptoms you describe and from a physical examination can confirm the diagnosis by running a variety of tests, including a blood test, an ultrasound, a urine analysis, an X-ray, or a urogram, in which a die is injected into the bladder to reveal stones unnoticed by an X-ray.

The treatment of kidney stones depends on their size and the location. Most stones can be treated without surgery by just flushing out the system—drinking two to three liters of water a day and staying physically active. If there's an infection associated with the blockage, you'll get antibiotics. Another available treatment is lithotripsy, in which a sound shock wave attempts to break up the stone to allow the crystals to discharge through urination. It's also possible to remove the stones surgically. You can go a long way to preventing kidney stones by eating a balanced diet, exercising, and drinking a lot of fluid, two to three quarts of water a day.

Gynecological Problems (For Women Only)

The more complicated the machinery, the greater the expertise necessary to fix anything that goes wrong with it. That's true for exotic cars as well as for some of the more exotic parts of the human anatomy. And so we have a branch of medicine known as gynecology, which specializes in treating the uniquely female parts of the human anatomy—the vulva, vagina, uterus, fallopian tubes, and ovaries. Any female of any age can have a gynecological problem, but as women get a bit older, some gynecological problems are more prevalent than others.

Vaginitis, an infection or inflammation of the vagina, is probably one of the most common conditions a woman can have. It's known by many names and is perhaps most often referred to as a "yeast infection." But many organisms can cause a vaginal inflammation, with yeast or *C. albicans,* being but one. Bacteria, parasites, and viruses can also trigger vaginitis, as can an allergic reaction or a hormonal change.

Normally the vagina is an area of the body where there is a balance of bacteria and yeast. But if you have a medical condition such as diabetes, or if you are taking medication such as antibiotics, then the balance of vaginal flora is altered; either the yeast or the bacteria becomes overgrown, and a vaginal infection occurs.

The symptoms of vaginitis include burning, itching, abnormal vaginal discharge, painful sexual intercourse, and painful urination. Most women with vaginal infections do not have any symptoms, however. By doing a physical examination, a doctor can diagnose vaginitis, which can then easily be treated with topical or oral medications.

Troubles related to menstruation are another source of common gynecological problems. One of these is *dysmenorrhea,* a painful menstruation that's usually due to a cramping of the uterus when bleeding occurs during the menstrual cycle. This can be seen as early as the teen years when a young girl begins to have her menstrual cycle, but for many women it only develops over time. It can last just a few hours or as long as several days. Other symptoms associated with dysmenorrhea include headaches, pelvic tenderness, back pain, diarrhea, and nausea, all of which can be attributed to the contractions of the uterus that occur during menstruation. For many women, the most effective treatments are simple pain relievers or sedatives. In severe cases, medication to decrease the amount of a biochemical called prostaglandins, which are produced during menstruation, relieves the pain.

PMS, or *premenstrual syndrome,* is a cluster of behavioral symptoms resulting from the hormonal changes that occur about two weeks before menstruation. The symptoms themselves appear right before or during menstruation. Up to 40 percent of women may be affected by PMS, though only 5 to 10 percent have a severe form that requires treatment. The behavioral symptoms involved range from depression, aggression, irritability, and anxiety to mood swings, nervous tension, and food cravings. And for many women PMS also includes headaches and fatigue. Because the problem is difficult to identify, treatment is problematic.

Dietary and other lifestyle changes can have a direct affect on PMS. Women who exercise regularly report having fewer PMS symptoms. Reducing salt in the diet can help minimize bloating and swelling, while reducing caffeine and alcohol can minimize irritability and mood swings. Yoga, meditation, and other relaxation techniques can help reduce the physical discomfort of PMS and lower stress. Calcium and moderate doses of magnesium and vitamin E may also be helpful in decreasing many PMS symptoms. Other treatments for PMS include anti-inflammatory drugs, such as ibuprofen to reduce PMS-associated pain, and diuretics, which may help reduce fluid buildup and decrease bloating.

Another common gynecological condition, *endometriosis,* affects about 20 percent of American women of childbearing age. The condition gets its name because it involves the endometrium, which is the tissue that lines the uterus. The tissue plays a major role in getting pregnant and is shed during menstruation. In endometriosis, cells from the endometrium migrate and become embedded outside the uterus or in the major muscle of the uterus. During menstruations, these out-of-place cells react the same way as the bleeding endometrium within the uterus; when these cells outside the uterus start bleeding, they can create excessive menstrual cramps and incredible pain. And if those cells are numerous, the bleeding can pocket and eventually form fibrous bands of scarlike tissue, which may create terrible pain during intercourse and block the fallopian tubes, causing infertility.

A gynecologist can diagnose endometriosis after reviewing a patient's history and performing a physical examination or, if necessary, doing a laparoscopy. In this procedure a small visual scope is inserted through a tiny puncture hole in the abdomen, providing a good view of the internal anatomy of the pelvis and any endometriotic sites that may be present. These sites can either be surgically removed or burned off. If the coverage is significant, other treatments like hormone therapy are recommended to try to disintegrate these tissues and encourage their reabsorption. A patient whose endometriosis is very severe may end up needing a *hysterectomy,* which is the surgical removal of the uterus and surrounding tissues.

A *uterine fibroid* is a tumor in the female pelvis. These are nodules of smooth muscle and connective tissue that grow within the wall of the uterus. They range in size from microscopic to ten inches and are more commonly seen in African American women than in white women. Although fibroids are very rarely associated with cancer, they can degenerate into cancerous lesions. Obesity has been linked to the development of fibroids, but the association is not a strong one.

Women who have fibroids, especially small ones, may not have any symptoms. If the fibroids are a little bit larger, women may complain of pressure, painful menstruation, back pain, excessive or heavy menstrual periods, frequent urination because of the pressure on the bladder, or painful intercourse.

Depending on the size and location of the fibroid and the age of the patient, treatment can range from nothing more than observation to a *myomectomy*, the surgical removal of fibroids, or a hysterectomy. There are new noninvasive procedures that women should consider, such as *embolization*, which involves blocking the vessels that feed the fibroid in an effort to shrink it, as well as *cryosurgery*, which is the freezing of fibroids.

Cervical Cancer

Cancer of the cervix is one of the most common cancers among women. The cervix is the lower part of the uterus, and it connects the upper part of the uterus, where a fetus grows, to the vagina, or birth canal. Nearly ten thousand women contract cervical cancer in the United States each year, and about four thousand die from it annually. It rarely occurs in women younger than twenty; half of women diagnosed with the cancer are between the ages of thirty-five and fifty-five.

Cervical cancer was once one of the most common causes of cancer death in American women, but the incidence of the cancer dropped by 74 percent during the second half of the twentieth century, thanks to the Pap test, a screening procedure that finds precancerous changes in the cervix.

Now at the dawn of the twenty-first century, there is still more good news in the battle against cervical cancer. With the FDA's 2006 approval of a new vaccine called Gardasil, cervical cancer may soon be a thing of the past. The vaccine, approved for girls and women from nine to twenty-six years old, is said to guard against 70 percent of cervical cancers and 90 percent of genital warts caused by human papillomavirus (HPV). The vaccine is expected to save thousands of lives in the United States and hundreds of thousands of lives worldwide.

Early Menopause

Some medical therapies, such as radiation treatments and chemotherapy, can lead to premature menopause (see "The Changes," page 193). So can a total hysterectomy, which is the surgical removal of both the uterus and the ovaries. One percent of women are affected by premature ovarian failure (POV); this is usually seen in women younger than forty years of age and is due to genetic factors or an autoimmune disease. POV has puzzled researchers for decades, and there is at present no safe and effective treatment for restoring the normal function of the ovaries.

Infertility

Infertility is a disease of the reproductive system defined as the inability to achieve pregnancy after one year of unprotected intercourse. It's a myth that if you try hard enough, pregnancy is guaranteed. Infertility is a medical condition.

One in seven couples experience infertility. Though it's often assumed that infertility is largely a female problem, the reality is quite different. About one-third of infertility cases are due to problems in the male partner, another third of the cases are due to the female partner, and the remaining third of infertility cases are unexplained. Male problems include conditions in which no sperm or too little sperm is produced. Conditions that affect women include ovulation disorders, blocked fallopian tubes (usually due to inflammation from infection or endometriosis), and anatomical deformities of the pelvic organ. While some people will insist that stress causes infertility, it is certainly true that infertility causes stress.

A diagnosis of infertility is made first by taking a thorough history and doing a physical examination, which are then followed by running a series of tests. For women, these include a laboratory test of hormone levels, ovulation charts, X-rays of the fallopian tubes and uterus, and a laparoscopy, in which a scope looks inside the body and provides a visual of the pelvic organs. Men usually have a sperm analysis. Eighty percent of the treatments for infertility fall into two categories—either medicinal or surgical. Several medicines are available that can improve ovulation, while surgical techniques can remove a blockage from the tubes and ovaries.

More aggressive treatments include artificial insemination and in vitro fertilization. With artificial insemination, ovulation is regulated with medications, and a health-care provider then artificially deposits semen in the vagina. For some patients, including same-sex partners, this is a very effective technique. In vitro fertilization is recommended for couples who want to conceive but are affected by a total blockage of the fallopian tubes or a very low sperm count. This technique surgically removes eggs from the ovary of the female and mixes an egg with sperm outside the body in a laboratory. Once a new embryo is formed, it is placed back inside the uterus. This technique has proven to be quite successful for couples who would otherwise not have been able to conceive on their own.

Twins and More!

If one is good, is two better? How about three? Or four? Or more? Of course, it's not exactly a matter of choice. Or is it?

The number of multiple births in the United States has increased dramatically over the past two decades. The number of twin births has increased by nearly 75 percent, making up 95 percent of the multiple births in this country, while the number of births involving three or more babies has gone up fivefold.

Two factors are responsible for this increase in multiple births. More women are waiting until they are over the age of thirty to have children, and these women are more likely to conceive multiples. The other, probably more significant factor, is due to the use of fertility-stimulating drugs and assisted-reproductive techniques (ART), such as in vitro fertilization. In fact, more than half of the infants born through ART were from multiple births.

The more babies a woman carries at once, the greater the risk of complications. The greatest risk with multiples is early labor resulting in premature births. More than half of twins, 90 percent of triples, and virtually all quadruplets or more are born preterm. These babies, like all preterm babies, face numerous health challenges both in the newborn period and later in life in the form of possible lasting disabilities. Other complications of multiples include high blood pressure and diabetes.

An ultrasound exam can detect almost all cases of multiples by the beginning of the second trimester. Because multiple pregnancies are automatically termed "high risk," it is absolutely essential that mothers-to-be of multiples eat properly, get plenty of rest, and make frequent visits to their doctor.

Joints—The First to Go

Arthritis comes in many unpleasant flavors, more than one hundred, in fact. But the most common is osteoarthritis, a disease that affects more than 20 million Americans and involves the gradual loss of cartilage in one or more of the weight-bearing joints. Cartilage, a substance made of protein, serves as a cushion between the bones of the joints of the spine, feet, hips, knees, and hands. Typically, osteoarthritis begins to develop after the age of thirty-five, more so in men than in women at that age, though after fifty-five more women than men are affected (see "Sports Injuries," page 156).

Osteoarthritis is just the natural aging process of the joints. With age, the water content of the cartilage increases and its protein content decreases, so that over time the cartilage becomes irritated and inflamed and eventually the joint degenerates. As the cartilage wears, the raw surface of the bones come into contact, causing friction, more inflammation, and more pain. The most common symptom of osteoarthritis is pain in the affected joint. The pain tends to get worse as the day goes by and may even be present when the joint is at rest. There may also be a swelling, warmth, or creaking of the joint. Over time the problem begins to limit the mobility of the joint itself.

Other conditions, besides this progressive aging process, can lead to early arthritis, however. Trauma, of course, can promote osteoarthritis, especially fractures or heavy falls. So can obesity. Because of the obesity epidemic among adolescents, teenagers, and young adults, the extra weight that we carry around puts a tremendous pressure on our joints when we reach our thirties and forties, and this ultimately leads to early osteoarthritis. One of the most common sites for osteoarthritis in adults is the knee because of the weight of all those extra pounds.

An X-ray is often sufficient to diagnose osteoarthritis. The X-ray may reveal either a narrowing of the space between the adjacent bones of a joint or perhaps the formation of bone spurs, which are outgrowths of new bone. But there are other diagnostic techniques, too. For instance, doctors can look inside the joint with *anthroscopy,* in which a tiny camera in a tube is inserted into the joint of the knee and enables the doctor to see exactly how much cartilage is left and what its condition is.

Since cartilage degeneration cannot be repaired, one of the pivotal treatments for osteoarthritis, especially if you're overweight, is weight loss. This will relieve a lot of the extra weight and burden on the skeletal system. Treatments aimed at alleviating the symptoms of this joint disease include anti-inflammatory medicines, physical therapy, and, if necessary, mechanical support devices. When these conservative approaches fail to control the pain, surgery has to be considered so that the surgeon can attempt to clean and restore the stress points in those joints as much as possible.

Many people with mild osteoarthritis turn to alternative medicine for help. Some people find the supplements glucosamine and chondroitin useful in relieving their pain and stiffness. Though manufacturers claim that these supplements help build cartilage, in reality there has been no proof that they do so. However, studies do confirm that glucosamine in particular can provide some relief of symptoms. Another effective supplement is omega-3 oil, which is naturally found in fish, though some people prefer to take fish oil capsules. By reducing inflammation, omega-3 oils can help with the symptoms of arthritis. Tylenol and nonsteroidal medications are often recommended for treating the pain associated with osteoarthritis.

The future is bright for the treatment of osteoarthritis. One surgical remedy on the horizon may involve removing some of the patient's own cartilage and growing more of it in a laboratory. The additional cartilage can then be reinserted into the splits that occur in the cartilage in the early phases of osteoarthritis, thereby creating a sort of patch for the joint. As promising as this new approach to an old problem may be, there is still

Sports Injuries

In the United States, sports injuries are now the number-two reason for visits to the doctor's office. Thanks in part to the medical advice that regular physical activity can help prevent everything from heart disease to diabetes, and motivated to achieve that prized, sculpted athletic look, more and more people are working out—often beyond the limits of their bodies for their age, unfortunately. For example, someone who has been jogging for fifteen years and begins to get knee pains, but keeps going, will eventually wear out the joint over time. Sometimes the problem is a matter of excess weight putting extra demands on the joints. Sometimes it's a matter of vanity. But with the common can-do, we-can-fix-that mentality that is so prevalent these days, and the improvements in surgical techniques over the past decade, more and more younger people than ever before are having knee and hip replacements, surgery for cartilage and ligament damage, and treatment for tendonitis, bursitis, and stress fractures. Don't let your exercise routine overrule common sense. Don't push your body beyond its limits.

To avoid the most common sports injuries, be sure to

- exercise regularly
- develop overall fitness (not just one part of the body)
- do warm-up exercises before any sport
- use protective gear when indicated
- play by the rules
- give your body time to recover after any exercise
- eat well and stay hydrated
- don't try to be Michael Jordan

nothing like taking a few preventative steps to hold osteoarthritis at bay. By watching your weight, eating a healthy and a balanced diet, and exercising regularly, you can really improve the overall quality of your skeletal system and therefore slow any early progression of osteoarthritis.

Rheumatoid Arthritis

The two most common types of chronic arthritis are osteoarthritis and rheumatoid arthritis. Rheumatoid arthritis affects only one-tenth as many people as osteoarthritis, which equals about 2 million people in the United States. Unlike osteoarthritis, rheumatoid arthritis is not a wear-and-tear disease. It is an autoimmune disease in which your own immune system attacks healthy tissue and causes inflammation that damages your joints.

Rheumatoid arthritis tends to attack the smaller joints—those in the hands and ankles, for example—rather than the larger joints such as the hips and knees. The symptoms are generally similar to osteoarthritis, though with rheumatoid arthritis the joint stiffness is worse in the morning or after prolonged activity, rather than getting progressively worse as the day goes by. Rheumatoid symptoms also tend to be symmetrical, in other words, affecting both hands, or both elbows, rather than one or the other as in osteoarthritis. Three out of four rheumatoid arthritis sufferers are women, while osteoarthritis strikes men and women about equally over time.

The aim of treatment in rheumatoid arthritis is to reduce the pain and inflammation; this is usually controlled through a variety of medications. Rest is important when the disease is active, while exercise is recommended when it's not so as to preserve strong muscles, flexibility, and joint mobility. Those with severe joint damage may require joint replacement surgery. Researchers are working hard to understand how and why rheumatoid arthritis develops, why some people get it and others do not, and why some people get it so much more severely than others.

Fibromyalgia

Pain is a sign of illness. It is a critical component of the body's defense system, and it is also very subjective. Some 90 million Americans suffer from pain of one sort of another. One type of pain now goes by the name of fibromyalgia, an arthritis-like condition that is characterized by generalized muscular pain and fatigue. Like many types of pain, fibromyalgia is an often misunderstood condition. People with fibromyalgia were once told that the condition was "in their head" because their lab tests were normal and their symptoms were so common.

Now fibromyalgia has been legitimized by the medical community, and it is diagnosed when you display the following symptoms: a history of widespread pain—on both sides of the body and above and below the waist—that is present for at least three months, and the pain is present in at least eleven of eighteen specific areas of the body (called tender point sites) when pressure is applied. These areas include the back of your head, upper back and neck, upper chest, elbows, hips, and knees. People with fibromyalgia also report headaches and facial pain; and a sensitivity to odors, noises, bright lights, and touch; and they often wake up tired even though they get plenty of sleep.

Fibromyalgia is thought to affect 3 to 6 million people in the United States, almost nine out of ten of whom are women. Doctors do not know what causes it. But those suffering a rheumatic disease, such as rheumatoid arthritis or lupus, are also more likely to have fibromyalgia. Treatment usually consists of a combination of medications—painkillers, antidepressants, and muscle relaxants—as well as relaxation and biofeedback techniques.

Multiple Sclerosis (MS)

MS? Those two letters are enough to send shivers up anyone's spine. But MS, or multiple sclerosis, is not always the debilitating disease we first think of when we hear those letters. That's no cause for celebration, of course, since there are still more than two hundred new cases diagnosed each week, adding to the three hundred thousand people living with MS in the United States today.

Multiple sclerosis is a chronic disease of the central nervous system, which comprises the brain, spinal cord, and optic nerve. The central nervous system sends and receives signals through a network of nerves that are insulated with a protective coating called *myelin*. MS basically strips the nerves of this protective coating in a process called *demyelination*. As a result, the nerve cells are not able to function adequately, and a disruption of the neurological messages sent through the central nervous system occurs. This can cause a variety of symptoms, some as mild as vision disturbances, dexterity problems, numbness, and tingling, to more severe ones such as complete blindness or paralysis.

MS is two to three times more likely to occur in women. When it strikes, MS can follow several different paths, though it's very unpredictable which particular path someone is going to follow. The most common is called relapsing-remitting MS, in which the symptoms flare up for a week or two and then diminish or disappear entirely before returning. This accounts for 85 percent of MS cases. Then there is primary progressive MS, in which the symptoms get progressively more severe over time. Secondary-progressive MS is a mix of the first two: the symptoms will come and go for a while, but then suddenly they return and get progressively worse. Relatively rare is progressive-relapsing MS, in which the symptoms worsen progressively, followed by periods of acute attacks.

Multiple sclerosis is often first diagnosed in people in their thirties, when the disease begins to create symptoms that are significant enough for those who are affected by it to seek out treatment. The symptoms of MS may begin as early as age fifteen, however, or as late as age sixty. The diagnosis is also often delayed due to the nature of the signs and symptoms. Multiple sclerosis is usually the last thing a primary care doctor will think about when faced with symptoms of fatigue, numbness, tingling, and visual disturbances; first on their minds will be anemia or the need for eyeglasses, for instance. A diagnosis of multiple sclerosis is finally made through a neurological exam conducted by a neurologist who specializes in MS and, usually, a CAT scan, which can show very clearly the MS lesions as bright spots in the cortex of the brain where this breakdown of myelin occurs.

The cause of multiple sclerosis is not known, and, to this day, there is no cure. But aggressive early treatment is now viewed as necessary and focuses on addressing the symptoms of the disease as well as on efforts to modify the number and severity of attacks and the progression of the disability. Steroids can shorten the duration of acute attacks by reducing the swelling and inflammation of the lesions in MS. Nontoxic chemotherapies can slow the progress of the disease and reduce the number of relapses by dampening the activity of the immune system. Several beta interferon products have also successfully decreased the relapse rate of MS, increased the time between attacks while reducing their severity, and decreased the total number of lesions.

Those with the milder forms of multiple sclerosis have found help through alternative therapies, though research has been inconclusive, and it is not regarded as the gold standard of care for MS. But acupuncture, for instance, which supposedly acts by adjusting the flow of energy through key points in the body, is said to relieve the pain related to MS. Others claim that bee venom therapy helps stimulate the immune system and reduce the inflammation associated with MS lesions. Hypnosis and tai chi, a form of mental and physical exercise, is also said to be effective in treating the pain associated with MS.

The bottom line is that even though MS is a progressive, degenerative disease of the central nervous system, it can be slowed down through proper treatment. Furthermore, people with MS can find incredible support systems, both through local groups and national associations, that provide information about the disease, organize activities, and fund re-

What Do Nancy Davis and Montel Williams Have in Common?

At the age of thirty-three Nancy Davis, a mother of five children, was diagnosed with MS. At that time, in 1991, there was very little information available on the disease, and there were no drugs on the market to help stop its progression. So Davis decided to commit herself to helping find the cause and a cure, and in 1993, she founded the Nancy Davis Foundation for Multiple Sclerosis. The foundation raises funds through its Race to Erase MS program, an annual celebrity gala benefit. All the proceeds go to the Nancy Davis Center Without Walls, a collaboration of physicians, scientists, and clinicians nationwide who are developing research programs and therapeutic approaches to eradicate MS.

The Emmy award–winning talk-show host Montel Williams was himself diagnosed with MS in 1999 and, like Davis, he decided to lend his time and talents to raising awareness of the disease, raising funds for research, and providing inspiration to others who have the disease. In 2000, he founded the Montel Williams MS Foundation to further the scientific study of this disease.

Today the public awareness of MS has grown tremendously. There are now five drugs that can slow the progression of the disease, and there are support and educational programs for MS victims around the country. Hopes are running high that this disease will one day be conquered.

search into MS. So a diagnosis of multiple sclerosis doesn't mean you should give up on life. Many people with MS have thriving and successful lives, and hopefully, in the very near future, we're going to find a cure for MS and eradicate this problem. (See "What Do Nancy Davis and Montel Williams Have in Common?," above.)

Looking Toward the Next Decade

Unless you've been thrown a loop with a genetic disease, you're now cruising in life. But there is good news and bad news ahead. The bad news is that you will never be as physically strong as you have been up to now, though if you follow the basics—eat well, exercise, and stay away from drugs, including cigarettes and alcohol—you can maintain a supremely healthy body. The good news is that you're getting smarter all the time. Much of that comes from simple experience. You've got four decades under your belt now. You know what to do in life. Go for it.

Test Checklist for this Decade

	Check BMI
	STDs/HIV tests
	Tetanus booster
	Gynecological exam (yearly)
	Dental cleaning (yearly)
	Cholesterol test (every five years, for men starting at thirty-five)
	Blood pressure check (every two years)
	Breast self-examination (monthly)
	Skin check (every three months)
	Baseline mammogram (for high risk women)
	Mental health screening (for depression, if needed)

The Cadillac Years

5

(The Fifth Decade: Ages 40 to 49)

You're finally starting to feel really comfortable in that body and mind of yours. Then suddenly you start feeling (how shall I say this nicely?) less than limber, and looking a little larger than you used to be, perhaps? Some little things—or some big things—are no longer working as they used to. And if you've been overdoing it for four decades, you're starting to see some major roadblocks up ahead.

Gynecolog
Dental Cl
Cholester
Blood Pr
Breast S
Bone De
Mamm
Skin Cl
Full Ph
Choles
Blood
Visio
STDs
Men
Check

M any people have an awakening at the age of forty. Suddenly they realize that they need to take care of themselves. These thoughts may be prompted by the need to take care of aging parents, or perhaps by an increased maturity that leads them to reevaluate the things that are truly important in life—like their health. In any case, many people in this decade will start to be more careful in watching what they eat to control their weight, take better care of their skin, and even, by gosh, start to exercise! It's a welcome insight because it's really never too late to start doing something good for yourself.

Dr. Manny's Freedom Diet Plan

One recent survey of Americans on body image found that more than half of all men and women would rather lose their job than gain an extra seventy-five pounds. And nearly 20 percent of the population would give up, or consider giving up, twenty IQ points to have the perfect body. Obviously weight and the way we are perceived is an important factor in our daily lives. It's not surprising then that dieting is on the minds of so many people these days, particularly as people get on in their forties, when the metabolism begins to slow and the pounds begin to add up. So which diet is best? I'll tell you.

First, let's look at some of the big blockbuster diets that have appeared over the past decade or so—the South Beach Diet, the Atkins Diet, the Mediterranean Diet, and so on. Each one of these diets has simply incorporated a different method of teaching you about nutrition in order to get you to lose weight. Each one gives you something to focus on, a behavior to motivate you, which is great because, after all, to lose weight you have to change your thinking. But if you look at the fundamentals, the underlying theme of each diet is calories. Whether you do Atkins, South Beach, or Dr. Phil, it's really all about calories.

When reviewed carefully, most diets are really nothing more than low-calorie nutrition plans disguised by clever marketing gimmicks. Scientific-sounding "facts" and hocus-pocus "research" are just ornaments on the diet tree. Diet-plan marketers go to great lengths to explain how their diet can work for everyone, or claim that it is carbohydrate intake or fat intake—or whatever the bad intake of the day is—that's the culprit. However, the bottom line is that the only way to lose weight is to have a caloric deficit, which occurs only when you burn more calories than you consume. The average American today consumes three hundred more calories per day today than did the average American of 30 years ago. Today's average American also burns 260 *fewer* calories each day due to increased automation, technology, and sedentary occupations. Put those numbers together, and it becomes rather obvious why America's waistline is growing at an alarming rate.

Check Your BMI

The BMI can tell you if you are underweight, normal, overweight, or obese. Adults twenty years old and older can calculate their BMI with this formula:

$$BMI = \frac{weight/pds}{height/in \times height/in} \times 703$$

You are UNDERWEIGHT, if your BMI is below 18.5.

You are of NORMAL WEIGHT, if your BMI is between 18.5 and 24.9.

You are OVERWEIGHT, if your BMI is between 25.0 and 29.9.

You are OBESE, if your BMI is 30.0 or more.

So here is Dr. Manny's Freedom Diet. If you really want to lose weight, you have to do two things: eat fewer calories *and* burn more calories. This is not an optional "either/or" plan but an "and" plan. Of course, the calories you eat should be healthy calories. That's all. Eat less. Exercise more. It really is that simple.

Fight obesity. Spread the word.

To Sweeten (Artificially)—or Not?

Let's face it, Americans love their sweets! That is why artificial sweeteners have assumed such an important role in our diets. We are not totally to blame. Madison Avenue has done a pretty good number on us over the years. But we should nevertheless be aware of certain facts about these products.

The most popular artificial sweetener these days is Splenda. Though labeled "natural" by the FDA, Splenda is not completely natural. Actually, it is partially synthetic (sucralose) and made up of two compounds, sugar and chlorine. The good news is that the digestive process absorbs chlorine poorly. The bad news is that chlorine can be deposited in fat cells and stay there for a long time. We really don't know yet what the long-term effects of this could be.

Aspartame, which is sold under the tradename NutraSweet or Equal, is another popular artificial sweetener. The FDA approved it in 1981 after tests showed it did not cause cancer in laboratory animals. But not all of the laboratory experiments agreed. Aspartame has had the most complaints of any food additive available to the public. A new seven-year study on aspartame found that the sweetener was associated with high rates of lymphoma, leukemia, and other cancers in rats that were given doses equivalent to five twenty-ounce diet sodas a day. I know people who live on that stuff, and you probably do, too.

Less well known is stevia, the "sweet herb." It has been used in South America for hundreds of years without ill effects, and it's the most popular sweetener in Japan. But there has never been a significant study on its safety, and it has not been approved by the FDA for use in the United States. However, stevia is much lower in calories than sugar, and its use is gaining momentum here in the States.

So which artificial sweetener should you use? When in doubt, go natural. That means the best solution is simply to decrease your dependence on sweets. Also bear in mind that you shouldn't be giving artificial sweeteners to kids at all.

Exercise

People spend an enormous amount of time trying to find the perfect exercise, and while they're doing that, their clock is ticking. Any physical activity is great, though the best kinds of exercise for you are those like walking, swimming, running, hiking, and skiing—all of which have a "global" impact on your body and mind. Most important, you should stick to the exercise of your choice and do it regularly. If you adhere to those two principles, you're going to burn calories, feel better, improve your metabolism, and benefit your health.

Any activity you do during the day—from climbing stairs, to housecleaning, to watching TV—will, of course, burn calories (see "Burn, Baby, Burn," page 169). But those activities don't provide the necessary continuity, and I think the essence of getting into shape and having a good metabolism has to do with a continuity of exercise. In other words, it's better to burn 120 calories a day, seven days a week, doing your favorite exercise, for example, than to burn 800 calories doing the housework once a week. It's the exercise *regimen* that has an impact on your health, not necessarily the intensity.

It is also very important to drink adequate amounts of fluid when you exercise. You need to drink about a half cup of water for every fifteen minutes of vigorous exercise. People think that muscle cramps during exercise

Burn, Baby, Burn

Estimated number of calories burned per minute based on an individual weighing about 150 pounds:

Sitting: 1

Talking on phone: 1

Sleeping: 1

Driving: 2

Housework: 3

Cooking: 3

Washing dishes: 3

Stretching: 4

Sex (active): 5

Walking (3 mph): 5

Calisthenics (moderate): 5

Ballroom dancing (fast): 6

Gardening: 6

Swimming (moderate): 7

Aerobics (low impact): 7

Hiking: 7

Jogging: 8

Stair step machine: 8

Bicycling (12 to 14 mph): 10

Basketball (full court): 12

Running (10 mph): 20

To easily calculate how many calories you burn in a day, go to www.healthstatus.com and click on "Calculators" then "Calories Burned."

are caused by a shortage of electrolytes, but that's not true. You get muscle cramps because of water loss and dehydration. Drink that water!

Doing It—or Not (Lack of Libido and Other Sexual Problems)

One reason—if not the main reason—we diet and exercise is that we want to look good to the opposite sex (or maybe the same sex). And, of course, one reason—if not the main reason—we want to do that is to be attractive to our (real or imagined) sexual partner. Now, what does any of this have to do with health, you wonder? The answer is, plenty. A healthy sex life improves your overall quality of life. It improves your immune system because it significantly relieves stress. Good physical exercise burns calories, and it improves your mood by pumping endorphins into your bloodstream that make you feel good. It also plays a key role in keeping couples together, so the benefits of sex are innumerable.

But once you get on into your forties, you might find your sex drive shifting into a lower gear. This diminished or lack of sex drive is more common in women than it is in men. Even men with erectile dysfunction (see "ED Education," page 172) usually have a normal sex drive. While libido problems can be either physical or psychological, the root causes tend to be the same in both sexes. Alcoholism is the main physical factor responsible for a decreased libido; another is drug abuse, of cocaine, for example. Obesity and anemia are other potential physical problems. And there are certain tumors of the pituitary gland that increase the hormone prolactin, which lowers the libido. Some prescribed medications, especially antidepressants, lower the level of the hormone testosterone, which is needed by both sexes to maintain an adequate sex drive. Psychological factors influencing libido include depression, stress, and confusions about sexual orientation.

Anyone with a lack of sexual desire should first try to take these factors out of the equation. So if you're drinking excessively, overweight, depressed, or taking medications, these issues need to be dealt with to resolve a flagging libido. Counseling can help with the psychological problems of sexual hang-ups, depression, or stress.

There is no magic remedy for the loss of sexual libido. Though testosterone has been identified as a key hormone that improves sexual appetite in women, doctors who have been giving women testosterone supplements for the past thirty years have found that it has little effect on their libido, while it sometimes causes facial hair growth, a deepened voice, and an enlargement of the clitoris. I have no doubt that one day there will be a libido pill for women and men, as I'm sure the drug companies are hard at work on this potentially lucrative solution.

There are a number of other sexual problems that women may experience at any age. One is *dyspareunia,* or painful sexual intercourse. Any part of the genitals can cause pain during sex, including the skin around the vagina. Vaginal infections, like yeast infections or viral infections, are a common cause, and the pain can be felt when either a tampon or penis is inserted into the vagina. It can also occur from just sitting or wearing pants. To treat dyspareunia, physicians may recommend hormone creams, dilators to help stretch the vagina, Kegel exercises, or, in rare cases, antidepressants.

Another potential cause of dyspareunia is *vaginismus,* an involuntary contraction of the vaginal muscles that may prevent insertion of the penis during intercourse. The diagnosis of vaginismus is usually problematic because it's often difficult to separate the physical pain with the emotional anxiety of experiencing that pain; in other words, just the fear of the pain can cause vaginismus. Any woman complaining of these symptoms should be taken seriously. A doctor must conduct a physical examination to eliminate the possibility of such physical causes as infections, fibroids, or anatomical deformities of the uterus, ovaries, or vagina. Even vaginal dryness can cause painful sex. A decrease in estrogen at menopause can cause the vaginal walls to become dry, creating a discomfort or pain during intercourse.

If there are no treatable physical conditions, it's important to discuss the woman's feelings as well as the physical situations that lead to this type of discomfort. Some women have a very positive attitude toward sex; other women have had negative sexual experiences that play a significant role in their fears and negative feelings about sex. Some women may have a history of sexual abuse, rape, or trauma, for instance; these things need to be identified in a very delicate way. Treatment of vaginismus usually involves practicing relaxation techniques and doing Kegel exercises to relax the vaginal muscles. At home, one exercise that may prove beneficial is to have your partner gradually insert a dilator into your vagina. This must be done at a pace with which you feel comfortable until the pain and discomfort are overcome. Partner, doctor, and patient all have to be in sync for this type of therapy to be successful.

Many women experience discomfort or pain at the time of their period. This pain is caused by contractions of the muscle of the uterus during menstruation that occur due to the release of the prostaglandins, which are hormones that are produced in the lining of the uterus. For most women these menstrual contractions are neither severe nor disabling. But some women experience significant menstrual pains called *dysmenorrhea*. Women suffering from dysmenorrhea should exercise, get plenty of sleep, and avoid stress. Over-the-counter painkillers can minimize the amount of prostaglandins released, and they usually help reduce the pain. If the painkillers are not effective, your doctor will have to look for other things that are causing the pain. And ultrasound is sometimes used in such cases to make sure you don't have any other medical conditions, like pelvic inflammatory disease, endometriosis, or fibroids.

E.D. Education

It used to be called impotence. But thanks to the proliferation of drug industry advertisements that now threaten to overwhelm our television programs, today we know it as erectile dysfunction, or, more discreetly, simply as E.D. Whatever you want to call it, though, it's the man's inability to achieve or maintain an erection sufficient to satisfy him or his partner during intercourse. When it occurs in young men, it's usually just a matter of momentary anxiety. In middle-aged men, it's often caused by stress, guilt, or overwork. In fact, most men experience it at some point in their lives by age forty, though usually only briefly, and they are not psychologically affected by it. But it gets more common with age, and for some men—as many as 30 million of them, according to the drug companies—it occurs frequently and causes serious emotional and relationship problems.

In many cases E.D. is due to the deterioration of the blood vessels that carry blood into the penis. A host of things can cause this deterioration, including nicotine, which narrows the blood vessels, excessive alcohol, and certain prescription drugs, notably antidepressants. Some physical problems can contribute to the deterioration, too, such as diabetes, high blood pressure, and obesity.

If you have difficulty getting an erection, get help. Discuss it with your partner, and consult your doctor, who will help you find the cause of your E.D. Treatment will, of course, depend on the cause. Though there are a number of mechanical devices that can help men get a better erection, including splints, rings, and pumps, it's the E.D. drugs that have revolutionized the treatment of this problem. They work well for most men, and if one drug doesn't work for you, try one of the others; but always work with a doctor's guidance since the drugs can have significant side effects.

Breast Cancer

The female breast is a remarkable collection of glands and fatty tissue that lies between the skin and the chest wall. Its main function is to produce milk for a baby. Inside this collection of glands are lobules where milk is produced. There are also blood vessels that feed into these glands, as well as lymphatic vessels that lead into the breast, making the breast a hyperdynamic structure of fatty tissues, glands, blood vessels, and lymphatic vessels. But the very things that make this structure so remarkable also make it highly danger-

Magic Pills

Three oral medicines for erectile dysfunction can improve a male's response to sexual stimulation: Viagra, Cialis, and Levitra.

Viagra was one of the first to hit the market in 1998, though it was first used as a potential treatment for angina. It works, usually within an hour, by widening the blood vessels. It lasts about four hours, but can be blocked by food in the stomach. It interacts with many medications and can cause headaches, vision problems, indigestion, palpitations, and dizziness, among other side effects.

Cialis works like Viagra and has similar side effects, and it can also cause back and muscle pain. It also interacts with other drugs, but is not blocked by food, and lasts twelve hours.

Levitra works like Cialis and Viagra, with similar side effects and drug interactions, but is not as long-lasting as Cialis.

ous when cancer occurs. When cells in the breast grow out of control and form cancerous tumors, they can easily and rapidly spread via those blood vessels and lymphatic vessels into nearby tissues and other parts of the body.

Every woman is at risk for developing breast cancer. About two hundred thousand cases are diagnosed every year, and it is second only to lung cancer in the number of deaths caused among American women annually. In terms of lifetime risk, that means that one out of eight women will develop breast cancer, and one out of twenty-eight will die from it. All women age forty and older are at risk for breast cancer, though most breast cancers occur in women over the age of fifty.

Some risk factors for breast cancer are avoidable. Taking birth control pills (see "The Pill and Breast Cancer," page 108) or hormone replacement therapy, not breast-feeding after having a child, having two to five alcoholic drinks a day, being overweight, and not exercising all increase the risk for breast cancer. But most of the factors that put a woman at risk for breast cancer are unavoidable. Getting older is one risk you can do nothing about. Being Caucasian is another. Having a family history of breast cancer in a sister or mother doubles your risk. The risk also increases if you had your first period before the age of twelve, had menopause after the age of fifty, or never had children. There are some genetic mutations, especially in Jewish families, such as the BRCA1 or BRCA2 mutations, which women may inherit from their parents, and which result in a 50 percent chance of getting breast cancer before the age of seventy.

Every effort is being made to prevent breast cancer. But since, unlike with lung cancer, there's no clear cause of breast cancer, all we can do right now is manage the risk factors. Avoid excess alcohol and long-term estrogen replacement therapy, watch your weight, exercise regularly, and, if you have a child, be sure to breast-feed. If you have a familial genetic predispositions based on the mutation of BRCA1 or BRCA2, or a history of breast cancer in the family, you can take certain drugs like tamoxifen or raloxifene, which have been found to be effective in preventing breast cancer. If your mother or sister had breast cancer, you should begin screening for the disease ten years before the age at which they were diagnosed. (If your mother got breast cancer at the age of forty-seven, for instance, you should begin screening at age thirty-seven.)

Screening tests for breast cancer are fundamental. The most important thing a woman can do to minimize her chances of getting breast cancer is to have regular mammograms, to learn how to perform breast self-examination, to actually perform the breast self-examinations, and to undergo regular physicals. The earlier the breast cancer is picked up, the more effective the treatment and the more curable the disease. Many times a mammogram can pick up a tumor before it is even felt. Women should get a yearly mammogram starting at the age of forty (earlier for those with a family history of the disease or a genetic mutation that increases the risk of breast cancer). Women between the ages of twenty to thirty-nine should have clinical breast exams at least every two to three years and then annually after the age of forty.

But don't depend entirely on the mammograms. About 15 percent of the tumors you can feel in the breast never appear on a mammogram. That's the reason why every woman should do a breast self-examination at least once a month. Once you become familiar with your breast, it should be easy to recognize any abnormality that occurs. The early stages of breast cancer are completely without

What to Expect at Your First Mammogram

The entire mammography exam, during which a medical technician takes two images of each breast, lasts about fifteen minutes. You will be asked to stand in front of the mammography machine and place your breast on a small platform. The technician will lower a plastic plate directly on top of the breast to compress it in order to get a clear view of the tissue. This is not normally painful, but it may be somewhat uncomfortable. (If you have very sensitive breasts, take acetaminophen or ibuprofen a half hour before your appointment.) The breast will be compressed for less than thirty seconds, as the machine releases the plate after each image. You will be asked to remain still and hold your breath while each X-ray is taken. Later that day a radiologist will interpret the images. If there are abnormalities, your doctor will contact you.

symptoms. But as a tumor grows in the breast, you might feel some lumps or very hardened areas of the breast or of the tissue underneath your arm, your breast might change in size as compared to the other, you might have some discharge from the nipple, the nipple might invert internally, or there might be some discoloration of the skin of the breast. While taken individually, these symptoms don't necessarily mean that you have breast cancer, they are all signs that should be brought to the attention of your doctor immediately.

Once breast cancer is suspected, whether it's on a diagnostic mammogram or otherwise, other tests will follow—usually a biopsy, because this

How to Do a Breast Self-Exam

1. Stand in front of a mirror, shoulders straight, hands on hips. Are your breasts evenly shaped, with no distortion or swelling? Do you see any redness or dimpling, or feel any soreness? Has your nipple changed position or been inverted? If so, tell your doctor.

2. Raise your arms, one at a time, and look for the same changes as in step 1.

3. Check for nipple discharge by gently squeezing each nipple between your thumb and index finger.

4. Now lie down and feel your breasts, using your right hand for your left breast and left hand for your right breast. With the first few fingers of each hand go over the entire surface area of your breast, feeling all of your breast tissue just underneath your skin and again deeper down with a firmer touch. If you locate any lumps or hard spots, notify your doctor.

5. Repeat step 4 while standing, perhaps while you are in the shower; it's easier to feel what's under the surface when your skin is wet and slippery.

is probably the only way to make sure you have or don't have cancer. Biopsies involve removing a small sample of the suspect tissue for further examination under a microscope by a pathologist. Not only do pathologists look for the cancer, they also seek to determine what kind of receptors—estrogen or progesterone—the cancer tissue has. The receptors help determine what type of therapy you will receive for the cancer; there are specific therapies directed at each type of receptor that improve the outcome.

The "stage" or location of the cancer is also determined during the diagnosis. If it's located in a lobule or duct of the breast, the cancer is at Stage 0. If the tumor is less than 2 centimeters but has not spread beyond the breast itself, it's Stage 1. Stage 2 involves tumors that are less than 2 centimeters and have migrated beyond the breast to the lymphatic nodes, or are greater than 2 centimeters and haven't spread outside the breast. Stage 3 involves more advanced breast cancers, greater than 5 centimeters, that have spread to the lymphatic nodes under the arm. Stage 4 is metastatic cancer, meaning that it has spread outside the breast to other organs.

Surgery plays a major role in the treatment by essentially removing as much of the cancer as possible. For the very early stages of breast cancer, the treatment is called a lumpectomy, which is the removal of the tumor and a little bit of normal tissue around the tumor. A lumpectomy is usually combined with radiation therapy. Partial mastectomies involve removing a larger piece of the breast. More advanced cancers are treated with modified radical mastectomies, meaning that the entire breast and the lymph nodes are removed. Most women who have total breast removal get reconstructive surgery in order to create a substitute breast mound. Those with high stages of cancer often also receive chemotherapy, with surgery or without surgery, in order to decrease the risk of the cancer's recurrence, though the side effects of chemotherapy can be considerable. Similarly, radiation therapy, which uses high-energy X-rays to kill cancer cells, is often used to reduce the risk of recurrence and to kill tumor cells that may be living in lymph nodes. Depending on whether the tumor expressed estrogen or progesterone receptors, patients may also receive hormonal therapy. Patients whose tumors expressed estrogen, for example, may receive an estrogen-blocking drug called tamoxifen for five years after their surgery.

Follow-up is very important for anyone who has been diagnosed with breast cancer. Women should be checked every three to four months. The longer they are free of disease, the better their long-term prognosis. After their five-year anniversary, they may need to see their doctor only once a year.

Take breast cancer seriously. It's a very deadly disease. But it's also very curable if caught early in the game.

Mental Health

The American family knows very little about mental health. In general, people are more informed about breast cancer than they are about mental illness. Nobody really wants to talk about it. And twenty years ago or so, the subject was strictly taboo. If you had a family member with a mental health problem, no one discussed it. People had a tendency to look at mental illness as a disability rather than a disease; they viewed it as a handicap. Folks with anxiety disorders, depression, and bipolar disorder thought better than to verbalize their problem, fearing they would be outcast or stigmatized because of it. Though the subject still raises eyebrows, mental health has lost some of its taboo stature of late.

Twenty percent of adults suffer from some sort of mental affliction, so there's nothing rare about it. If you look at its impact on our work force, mental health ranks as the second leading cause of people's inability to be fully productive in their jobs and in their careers. (Number one is heart disease; number three is cancer.)

The good news is that mental health diseases are often easily diagnosed and can be effectively treated. The bad news is that only one-third of the people with a diagnosable mental disorder gets the help they need. Why? Some people feel too embarrassed about the subject to seek help. Others don't know where to get help. Truth be told, mental health doesn't get much attention in our society. That subject goes to the bottom of the pile in terms of the number of the dollars it receives for research and the number of clinics that are available to treat people. Financially speaking, mental health is always the first to get the axe. It's poorly reimbursed by insurance companies, and for medical centers it's not at all cost effective; it's easy to see why. It takes much longer to treat a mental health patient than any other kind of patient. You can't see ten mental health patients in an hour. (And you actually have to have a conversation with them!)

The way we look at mental diseases has changed considerably over the last twenty years. One of the first breakthroughs came in 1952, when there was a national consensus among mental health professionals about how mental disorders should be classified, what the different categories are, and of what specific signs and symptoms each disorder consists. They issued a book of mental disorders called the *Diagnostic and Statistical Manual (DSM)* that pretty much spelled out what anxiety disorders are, from depressive disorders to manic depression to bipolar disorders to schizophrenia. The book gave clinicians a template from which to work and allowed them to make diagnoses on which they could all agree.

Mental health problems are believed to be the result of a combination of factors. Major depression, schizophrenia, and bipolar disorder seem to run in families, so there is clearly a genetic component to these problems. There are also developmental or environmental factors involved in mental health, such as childhood traumas, emotional scarring, and improper upbringing. But generally, mental disorders have a biological component as well, with the biology of the brain being a focal point. This realization led researchers to look closely at the biochemistry of the brain, and much progress has been made in understanding the biochemical mechanisms of thought processing, moods and hormones, and neurotransmitters such as serotonin and tryptophan. This spurred the creation of medications that targeted the deficiencies in the biochemistry of the brain, which has had a tremendous impact on the whole mood and psychology of the individual. We know more today than ever about how the brain works and how it affects our overall health.

But in our newfound reliance on pills as a solution to mental disorders, we have lost some of our ability to deal with the emotional consequences of these diseases. We'll prescribe pills for depression, for example, but we fail to recognize that there is a psychological component, a therapeutic component, that needs to be followed up on; people remember what they went through, how they felt, how they acted, and what impact the disease had on them. Regardless of how wonderful it can be, medication is not sufficient for mental disorders; we need more psychological counseling.

Nutrition also plays an important role in mental health. Because the brain is derived directly from food, what we eat has a direct impact on how it works—or doesn't work. Just like the heart and liver, the brain is an organ that is very sensitive to what we eat and drink. To remain healthy, the brain needs a balance of complex carbohydrates, essential fatty acids, amino acids, vitamins, minerals, and water. An improper balance of fatty acids, for instance, has been associated with depression and other mental health problems. Vitamins and minerals help improve mental functioning through their role in the brain's conversion of amino acids into neurotransmitters, which control our moods. Antioxidants are important for mental health as well because they tend to remove what I like to call the "biological debris" that can be toxic to normal cell function. A balanced

Is It the Violence?

Although there is a better understanding of mental illness today, the stigma persists. Why? Surveys suggest that the answer is a fear of violence. People with mental illness are perceived as more violent. But are they really? There is a greater risk of violence among individuals with a mental disorder who also have a substance abuse problem. And there is a slightly elevated risk for violence among people with a severe mental disorder who are not taking their medication. But it turns out that the risk of violence from mentally ill individuals is lower if they are strangers rather than family members. So there is very little risk of harm from casual contact with strangers who have a mental disorder. Who is to blame for this entrenched fear of violence from the mentally ill? The media is at least partly responsible, because they selectively cover stories that reinforce people's stereotypes linking violence to mental illness. Combine that with the fact that almost half of all Americans admit to knowing little to nothing about mental illness, and it's clear that more knowledge about the problem can only help reduce the stigma that still exists.

diet can help stabilize a person's mental state and can help minimize aberrations in behavior.

Bipolar Disorder

The prevalence of bipolar disorder (also known as manic depression) is now widely recognized by mental health professionals. Bipolar disorder is one of the complex depressive illnesses that affect both men and women equally. Although we have an understanding of its biochemistry, nobody really knows why it happens. Is it genetic or the result of life experiences and stress?

Bipolar disorder is composed of two mood changes. The first is depression—you're unhappy, lacking in interests and confidence, unable to enjoy things or to make simple decisions; and you're always tired, agitated, and irritable. You may even have suicidal thoughts. Many people with these symptoms, especially if they are mild or perceived to be mild, will find that the problem goes away by itself. But if the symptoms last longer than three to four weeks, you will need to seek help. Usually this will involve a course of antidepressant therapy like Prozac for about six weeks.

The manic phase is completely different. It is a reversal and exaggeration of the other symptoms. Now you feel incredibly happy and excited. You get irritated when people don't share your optimism, you're full of energy, and you can't sleep because you're so euphoric. You perceive everything as more important than usual. You might exhibit reckless behavior, overspending or making rash decisions. And you certainly are less inhibited by your sexual behavior. If these symptoms are persistent, you need to be on antipsychotic medication.

Once you've been diagnosed as manic depressive, taken the medication, and had some follow-up counseling or psychotherapy, you need to step back and ask yourself a couple of questions: "What did I learn from

How You Can Help

How do you deal with people who have a mental disorder? For those with depression, first and foremost, you need to understand them and be patient with them. But it is often very difficult to understand what depressed individuals want when they are pessimistic about everything. You have to realize that what is important is not so much what they are saying, as the way they're saying it. You can help by offering practical advice. Make sure that they can take care of themselves, that they're not becoming dysfunctional—sleeping twenty hours a day, not eating, not cleaning themselves. Certainly, if there's any hint they're thinking of harming themselves, you have to take them seriously and seek medical attention immediately.

When people are manic or in the manic phase of manic depression, you should avoid feeding into their euphoria. Try to minimize their exposure to parties and other gatherings; these situations will usually encourage their euphoric state and may lead to hostility, suspiciousness, and physically explosive behavior. Be careful not to engage them in an argument because they might have an outrageous point of view and a very aggressive way of presenting it. Manic depressives feed on confrontation. If a situation becomes explosive, get professional help immediately. Manic depressive people may sometimes need a short hospital admission to protect them from trouble.

this experience? What got me there?" Often when you think about it, you can figure out how you got to be that way. Once you have identified those causative factors, you can say, "Okay, now I'm going to do something about it."

One thing you can do something about is stress. If you have a tendency to be depressed or manic, or manic-depressed, you have to work on your stress. Avoid stressful situations and incorporate a lifestyle that allows you to avoid stress. Balance your life with work and other activities that can help you tone down your stress. You can do that by seeing a psychologist, by practicing yoga, meditation, or tai chi (a form of yoga and meditation combined), or by doing regular exercise. Also, evaluate your relationships with people. Relationships are a complex matter, whether you're talking about a friend, a spouse, or another family member. Take a close look at your relationships and ask yourself if they are, at the end of the day, hurting you because, again, you are going to need the support of the people around you to help you solve your mental health problem.

Streeeeeess

Stress is our body's ability to respond to our surroundings—how we react to our family, our work, and various events in our lives. Stress is normal. Everyone is under some kind of stress—every day. But there are two kinds of stress: the good and the bad. Good stress can be something like getting a new job or buying a first home. Bad stress can range from experiencing a difficult financial situation to having a sick family member to missing a flight to getting a flat tire in the pouring rain.

Short-lived stress rarely affects long-term health. But stress becomes a problem when it's chronic and difficult to identify. Stress manifests itself through feelings of sadness, anxiety, anger, frustration, guilt, or excitement. Our mood starts to fluctuate. Some people drink or smoke; others opt for healthier outlets such as jogging. Some just go shopping. Eventually, our body starts to ache here and there, first a little bit, then more and more. Those may seem like "phantom aches" at first, but as time goes by, they can become legitimate physical health threats. If left unchecked, stress can ultimately cause blood pressure oscillations and weaken the immune system, which makes us much more susceptible to illnesses that our body, under normal circumstances, would be able to fight. People can eventually die from the effects of stress because, at the end of the day, those under stress are going to have more heart disease, more diabetes, more obesity, and more gastric problems like ulcers than people who are relatively stress-free.

One of the most severe types of stress is called post-traumatic stress disorder, or PTSD. PTSD is a psychiatric disorder that occurs after experiencing an extremely stressful situation or witnessing a life-threatening event, like a terrorist attack, a violent personal assault, or a natural disaster. People suffering from PTSD have symptoms that include flashbacks, difficulty sleeping, mood changes, depression, and the inability to deal with everyday life. These are not those nutty people walking around in ripped and filthy clothes, talking to themselves and their imaginary friends. They are fully functional people, people like you and me, who may be stressed out by the daily media reminders of kidnapped children, serial killers, and sexual abuse. And oftentimes, these people don't even know they have PTSD.

It's important that you take stress seriously and learn how to handle it. First, recognize the signs and acknowledge them. Second, ask yourself: Am I leading a healthy life, exercising, not abusing drugs, including cigarettes and alcohol? If not, you have to make some lifestyle changes. The solution, many times, is right in front of you. But for the most part, if you recognize stress as something that is out there, and if you're able to manage it adequately, it will have no dire effects on your health. It is only when you ignore it and it becomes chronic and unstoppable that you need to seek professional help.

Signs of Stress

- Do you tend to race through the day, do everything yourself, and set unrealistic goals?
- Do you make a big deal of everything, blow up easily, and get angry when kept waiting?
- Do you frequently neglect your diet, exercise, and your sleep?
- Do you lack close, supportive relationships outside your family?
- Do you often fail to see the humor in situations that others find amusing?
- Do you ignore symptoms of stress and have no time for questions like this?

If you answered yes to most of these questions, chance are you are STRESSED OUT. Do something about it.

The Silent Killer

Hypertension is known as the silent killer for good reason. Some 50 million Americans have high blood pressure and one-third of those don't even know it, despite the fact that it's very easy to diagnose. Hypertension kills some forty thousand Americans each year, and another two hundred thousand die annually of a high-blood-pressure-related illness. People with hypertension are seven times more likely to have a stoke, six times more likely to have congestive heart failure, and three times more likely to develop a heart attack. In all, hypertension claims more lives per year in the United States than cancer. Those numbers are doubly sad: first, because they are so high, and second, because they could easily be so much lower. More than half of the people with hypertension are not receiving treatment at all, and one-quarter of them are being inadequately treated. Only about one-fifth are receiving the proper treatment to control their blood pressure.

There are two types of hypertension. More than 90 percent of all cases of hypertension involve what is known as essential hypertension, which is high blood pressure without a definite cause. The rest, fewer than 10 percent of the cases, have a known cause; this is known as organic hypertension, or secondary hypertension. Organic hypertension occurs when a specific disease, such as a tumor of the kidneys, vascular disease, or hormonal disease, causes your blood pressure to be elevated.

When we talk about blood pressure, we are referring to a comparison of the blood pressure when the heart is beating versus the pressure when the heart is resting. A blood pressure reading is represented as the *systolic* (or beating pressure) over the *diastolic* (or resting) pressure. A normal blood pressure is anything lower than 120 over 80. But if you are 140 over 90 or above, you have high blood pressure. Anything in between the two sets of numbers is considered prehypertensive.

How can you tell you have high blood pressure? Certainly not by your symptoms; most people with hypertension don't have any. But any qualified health professional can measure your blood pressure in a very non-evasive way using a blood pressure machine. Of course, if your blood pressure is very high, you will have symptoms like nose bleeds, irregular heartbeats, headaches, and dizziness.

Hypertension affects more males than females and more blacks and

Latinos than whites. The lifestyle characteristics that can put you at risk of developing hypertension include obesity, lack of exercise, a diet rich in sodium, and excessive alcohol consumption. Smoking raises blood pressure as well. Genetic factors may be involved, too, as some individuals have a family history of hypertension. In younger women, hypertension is sometimes associated with birth control pills. Other medications that can give you high blood pressure include some nonsteroid anti-inflammatories, cold remedies, decongestants, and appetite-suppressant pills.

Your diet plays a very significant role in blood pressure. Foods high in cholesterol thicken the blood with fat, and that forces the heart to work harder, thereby raising your blood pressure. As the heart works harder to push that blood through, the heart becomes larger because it has to expand more to grab enough volume in order to squeeze the blood out of its chambers. If the heart has to work harder, the heart and the arteries come under tremendous pressure and stress, and this, of course, weakens the heart. It also means that organs like the kidneys and eyes and liver don't get enough oxygenated blood, which causes cell damage to those organs that ultimately damages them.

A high salt intake also makes you retain more water in your vascular system, and that, too, increases your blood pressure. To reduce your risk of high blood pressure, the American Heart Association (AHA) suggests that you ingest no more than 2,400 milligrams of sodium a day. That's just one and a quarter teaspoons of salt per day, and it mounts up faster than you think; *many* foods, especially prepared foods, contain large amounts of sodium. And then there is all the salt we actually add to our food.

Being overweight is also a fundamental factor in developing high blood pressure. Conversely, losing weight is one of the essential ways of improving your blood pressure. Lack of exercise and physical inactivity is another risk factor for heart disease. This means that exercising will improve your cardiac performance, making your heart work better, thus lowering your blood pressure. Stress has also been linked to hypertension: it narrows the blood vessels, thereby causing high blood pressure, so it is vital for people who have high blood pressure to learn how to manage their stress.

The treatment of high blood pressure involves making dietary changes, losing weight, lowering cholesterol, practicing relaxation and meditation techniques, and getting some exercise. If these don't work, there are medications that can specifically target the kind of hypertension you have.

So how do we prevent high blood pressure? Number one, watch your weight. If you are 30 percent above your ideal body weight, you've got a problem and are more likely to develop high blood pressure. Second, if you're drinking excessively—more than three hard drinks a day—this also is a problem. Also, watch your salt intake; eat fewer processed foods. If you go out to eat, ask your wait person if the kitchen can reduce the amount of salt in your order. Eat a balanced diet. Consume foods that can help lower your cholesterol, like vegetables and grains. Don't smoke; nicotine is a major vasoconstrictor. And exercise regularly; try to do thirty minutes' worth of aerobic activities three to four times a week.

The bottom line on hypertension is to do your best to prevent it. If you can't, identify it, and then treat it. Whatever you do, don't become a statistic like so many other Americans.

Testing, Testing

Many people avoid going to the doctor unless they absolutely positively have to go. But beginning at the age of forty, many people start feeling a little something here, a little weakness there, and they'll at least start thinking about going for a checkup. You should do that; it's a good idea. In fact, between the ages of forty and fifty, you should have a full physical exam every one to five years. Have your cholesterol checked every five years. Get your blood sugar tested every three to five years. Have your blood pressure checked for hypertension, stroke, heart disease, and kidney damage every two years. Get an eye exam every couple of years. And have a skin check and dental checkup every year. In addition, women should have a Pap test, mammogram, and pelvic exam every year or so.

Unless there is a revolutionary breakthrough in medicine in the near future, chances are you have by now entered the second half of your life. Our bodies are essentially mechanical devices just like cars. Things break down; it's inevitable. So it's better to have yourself checked out and get things fixed before they leave you stranded in the middle of nowhere.

The Big Five-oh

Coming up is a numerical stumbling block that's largely psychological. There is probably no more depressing birthday than your fiftieth. But don't let it get you down. Just let it serve as a reminder to watch your health a little more closely than you have in the past. And if that number doesn't jog you into action, your body probably will, as it will be undergoing some subtle, and maybe not so subtle, changes in the next decade. You might try to ignore them, but you'll be better off dealing with them. I'll give you some tips on how best to ease through this next decade of life like a hybrid car in the middle of an oil crisis.

Test Checklist for this Decade

Check BMI
Tetanus booster
Gynecological exam (yearly)
Dental cleaning (yearly)
Cholesterol test (every five years, also for women beginning at age forty-five)
Blood pressure check (every two years)
Breast self-examination (monthly)
Bone density test
Mammogram (every one to two years)
Skin check (every three months)
Full physical (one to five years)
Cholesterol check (for women, every five years, starting at age forty-five)
Blood sugar check (every three to five years)
Vision check (every two years)
STDs/HIV tests
Mental health screening (for depression, if needed)

Keeping Up
with the Joneses

6

(The Sixth Decade: Ages 50 to 59)

"Changes, changes," goes the pop song.
And, indeed, with this decade come
some changes for both women and men,
some sneaking up on us, some sudden, even
as we plow ahead in life. We'll fight these
changes, of course, with a sports car or some
nip and tuck. But it's not the Joneses that
really matter, it's the Hormones.

The sixth decade of life is a time of transformation. For women the changes are usually summed up with the word "menopause." Men also seem to have a "pause" of their own during their fifties, even if it's not quite as obvious as it is for women. The changes in the body and mind caused by aging are now more obvious than in the previous decade, with graying hair, more wrinkles, and some memory lapses, perhaps, but the physical or intellectual activity of healthy fifty-year-olds is nothing to sneer at. It's worth noting that most of the men who became president of the United States have done so while in their fifties. And presidential aspiration is no better example of the wanting-to-do-it-all desires of this age group, whether those doing the desiring are men or women.

If there is a watchword for this decade, it's "hormones." Hormones exert a profound influence over our lives, though it's not until the fifties—when women begin to lose estrogen and men begin to lose testosterone—that we realize how important hormones really are to our health and well-being. The hormones produced by our body are responsible not only for reproduction, development, and normal behavior, but for the maintenance of our normal body processes as well.

The Changes

When people think about menopause, they often think about that old cliché—"the change." Menopause is not a single event, however, but a transition that begins in your forties, and continues into your fifties and sixties. By definition, a menopausal woman is one who hasn't had a period in twelve consecutive months, but menopause is actually a normal, biological process involving hormonal changes that results in both physical and psychological changes. It's not an illness, and it's not the end of your sexuality or your youth. In fact, many women feel that their lives actually *begin* at menopause.

The first indication that menopause is approaching is having irregular periods. They might stop for a couple of months, then get lighter, and eventually cease entirely. Along with that, of course, comes a decrease in fertility; ovulation begins to fluctuate and ultimately stops, though up until the moment you haven't had a period for one year you can still become pregnant. Vaginal changes occur as your ovary-produced estrogen levels decline; the tissues lining the vagina and the urethra become thinner and drier, which may lead to burning, itching, and an increased risk of bladder and vaginal infections.

Three out of four women report having troublesome symptoms during menopause, though their severity and frequency vary from one woman to another. Many women experience hot flashes as their estrogen level begins to drop; this drop causes the blood vessels to expand rapidly and the skin temperature to rise. Humid weather, confining spaces, spicy foods, and caffeine or alcoholic drinks can all trigger hot flashes. Some women entering menopause begin to have sleep disturbances, at least partially because of these hot flashes, or night sweats. The lack of sleep may eventually affect their mood and overall health.

Menopause may also produce a change in appearance. Some women gain weight when they become menopausal, usually an average of five pounds or so. There may also be a thinning of the hair, more wrinkles, and a loss of fullness in the breasts. With the drop in estrogen levels, the small amount of testosterone still produced by the body may lead to the development of some facial hair as well as hair on the chest and abdomen.

It's a good idea to pay a visit to your doctor as you begin to enter menopause so that you can start keeping a close watch on your hormone levels.

You want to do this for several reasons. One, menopause and the decrease of estrogen that comes with it puts you at greater risk for cardiovascular disease. That means you need to monitor your blood pressure more carefully, not smoke, and eat low-cholesterol foods to make sure that the natural aging process doesn't further increase your risk of heart disease. Another reason is that you will lose some bone mass, especially in the first couple of years of menopause. This makes menopausal women more susceptible to hip and other fractures, so it is important to make sure that you are taking adequate amounts of calcium. You'll need about 1,500 milligrams of calcium and about 400 to 800 international units of vitamin D per day from now on. You should also be exercising to improve the strength of your ligaments and your muscles around your bones in order to compensate for that loss of bone density. And because the vaginal mucosa gets thinned out due to the loss of estrogen, the bladder tends to protrude into the vaginal wall; as a result, many women will begin reporting symptoms of bladder dysfunction.

There are many things you can do to better adapt to menopause. For vaginal discomfort and dryness, use lubricants like KY Jelly and moisturizers. To optimize sleep, avoid drinking too much coffee or ingesting other sources of caffeine, especially during the first few years of menopause, because your body is changing so much. It's very important to develop relaxation techniques to deal with the stress. Exercise regularly, and do your Kegel exercises to improve the muscles in the vagina. Watch what you eat, watch your caloric intake, and take vitamin D and calcium supplements as needed. And don't smoke.

Serious symptoms of menopause may require medication, but what used to be standard hormone replacement therapy is no longer recommended (see "Hold the Hormones," page 196). Antidepressants, like Zoloft or Prozac, can be quite effective in dealing with mood changes. Women with very serious hot flashes may need a drug like Clonidine, a blood pressure medicine available in pill or patch form, to control the problem.

Nonhormonal medications such as Fosamax and Actonel are quite commonly prescribed today to treat osteoporosis or bone loss. These medications, whose primary side effect is gastrointestinal pain, have basically replaced estrogen as the primary mechanism to help women deal with osteoporosis in menopause. There are also specific vaginal estrogens—administered locally in ring, tablet, or cream form—that can significantly reduce vaginal dryness.

Some complimentary medicines are said to be quite effective in relieving menopausal symptoms. Natural estrogens called *isoflavones* can be

Hold the Hormones

Not long ago it was standard medical practice to give menopausal women hormonal replacement therapy (HRT). The therapy followed the standard medical practice of restoring what the body fails to produce on its own. Just as we replace insulin when the body doesn't produce enough of it, it seemed logical that we should be replacing estrogen when a woman's body was no longer producing enough of it.

Then the Women's Health Initiative (WHI) came along and published a study showing that estrogen therapy causes an increased risk of breast cancer and other diseases. So while estrogen therapy had helped prevent bone loss, it was also increasing the number of breast cancers and strokes in women. The estrogen in HRT came from horse urine, and when it was synthesized in the human liver, it would break down into two kinds of estrogen, the good estrogen a woman needs, and a bad estrogen that poses a health risk. For good reason, once these findings were released, millions of women stopped taking HRT.

Since 2002 many American women and their doctors have found an alternative treatment in what is called the bio-identical hormone approach. In contrast to traditional hormone treatment, bio-identical hormones are an exact match to the hormones produced naturally by a woman's body. Not only can they can be created by modifying soy or yam hormones (no more horse urine), but any molecule that does not exist on the human hormone counterpart is removed. While more studies on bio-identical hormone therapies are needed, a large body of evidence points to the potential advantages of this approach in the future.

found in certain foods like soybeans, chickpeas, and other legumes, while those known as *lignans* occur in whole grains, nuts, seeds, and beans. The Chinese, who have a diet rich in these types of foods, report fewer menopausal signs and symptoms, though there are no clinical studies to back up these claims. Vitamin E is also said to provide some mild relief for hot flashes. A very popular herb called black cohosh, which is used extensively in Europe for treating hot flashes, is becoming popular in the States, though again there are no major scientific studies to back up these reports. Other products like licorice, evening primrose oil, and wild yam are all said to be beneficial for menopausal symptoms. But before using any herbal treatments or dietary supplements, make sure you first get an okay from your primary care doctor, because many of these products can trigger allergic reactions or can cross-react with a prescribed medication you happen to be taking.

"Machopause"

Women are not the only ones who suffer from the effects of changing hormones. It can happen to men, too. Andropause, as it is known, is the male version of menopause. Just as estrogen is vital to females, testosterone is vital to the development and normal functioning of males.

If a man is healthy, his hormone production may remain normal into old age, and he may be able to produce sperm well into his eighties or even later. On the other hand, as men get older, starting usually between the ages of forty-five and fifty, subtle changes in the functioning of their testicles may take place that dramatically reduce their testosterone, with levels of the hormone dropping off more quickly in some men than in others. Typically, this decrease in male testosterone leads to symptoms of depression, fatigue, and lack of energy. In some men it may decrease their appetite for sex. A decline in testosterone can also put men at risk for heart disease and osteoporosis.

Andropause is more gradual in men than menopause is in women. It may also be accompanied by a variety of psychological effects known as a "mid life crisis," which is expressed through the purchase of a sports car, for instance, or through leaving their family and finding a younger woman. However, such behavior cannot be entirely explained by a drop in testosterone—usually there are other factors involved as well.

Though andropause has not been as well described in men as menopause has been in women, it's real, and it's clear that men do experience it. However, since the symptoms of depression and fatigue have traditionally been attributed to the aging process, andropause has not been recognized as a clinical problem and is still being debated. Consequently, you won't find many men going to see their primary care doctor saying, "I think I'm going through male menopause."

There are now diagnostic tests that can measure the amount of free or bioavailable testosterone in the body. You might think that hormonal replacement therapy for males would be an easy solution to the problem, but it isn't. Testosterone is a very strong hormone, and high levels of testosterone have been linked to heart disease and prostate cancer; so in the management of andropause, it's a good idea to look at factors that might influence the natural testosterone level of the individual without having to take in extra testosterone.

One such factor is obesity. If you are excessively overweight, the fat is going to interfere with your testosterone production, especially if that weight gain is the result of what I call the White Diet, which consists of white bread, flour, refined carbohydrates, and sugars. But by losing weight and decreasing your body fat, you can not only reduce your natural estrogen (yes, men have the female hormone in their bodies, just as females have the male hormone testosterone), but increase your natural level of testosterone as well. Many times this is all that is needed to overcome obesity.

Male hormonal therapy *is* an option for increasing testosterone levels, but it has to be very carefully monitored by an endocrinologist who knows how to prescribe testosterone: it's not only a question of *which* testosterone to give but *how much* to give. Other medications have been tried with some success, including Clomiphene, a medication that typically has been given to women to improve ovulation. In men, Clomiphene improves the natural levels of male testosterone by reducing their natural level of estrogen.

The best way to cope with andropause is to relieve your stress, eat a nutritious, low-fat, high-fiber diet, get plenty of sleep, exercise regularly, and limit your consumption of alcohol.

Healthy Metabolism

Creating a healthy metabolism is the key to preventing hormonal imbalance, particularly in our fifties. In fact, some physicians believe that many of the symptoms of menopause, for instance, may largely be due to a combination of poor diet, unhealthy lifestyle, and environmental pollutants. To back up such claims, they note that menopause in nonindustrialized countries is usually a gentle, barely noticeable process, whereas the symptoms of hormonal imbalance in Western cultures are often more significant and epidemic.

Diet, of course, plays an important role in our metabolism. Essential for normal hormone production and upkeep is a diet that is rich in whole grains, leafy greens, and other vegetables and fruits. If your diet is full of fast foods and trans-fatty acids, you are not getting the antioxidants, vitamins, and minerals you need in order to neutralize the effects of both the harmful environmental hormones to which you are exposed and the harmful by-products of our own metabolism. We are ex-

> **Metabolism** is a term derived from the Greek word for "change." When we talk about metabolism, we are referring to the various processes our body uses to convert food and other substances into energy and other products our body needs to maintain itself, repair damage, heal injury, and rid itself of toxins.

posed to a host of environmental hormones in our daily lives—from carpet glue to plastics to car exhausts to Styrofoam; these are absorbed by our system and cause harmful side effects.

Exercise also improves hormone functionality and metabolism. A sedentary lifestyle will slow down our metabolism, meaning that we retain more fat, which reduces the levels of estrogen and testosterone in our bodies. Chronic stress is a major cause of hormonal imbalance; it doesn't allow our adrenal glands to do their regular maintenance work because stress puts them in a constant state of alert. Finally, proper sleep is essential to keeping your metabolism balanced and your hormones in check.

Sleep is the time of your life when your body heals itself naturally. If you're sleep-deprived, if you don't get your eight hours at night, you are putting a serious strain on your hormone production and your body's ability to repair itself. Some doctors will go so far as to say that 90 percent of our waking health is dependent on our sleep.

So it is important when you get into this decade that you have your hormones tested when you go for your physical. It's just a simple blood test. So do it.

The Storage Sack (Gallbladder)

Unlike the heart or the lungs, the gallbladder is one of those organs about which people know next to nothing. And no wonder, the gallbladder is little more than a storage sack. What it stores is bile, which is produced by the liver. So what's bile? Bile is a substance that contains the enzymes needed to help break down the fat in our food. As we digest our food, the gallbladder excretes bile through the bile ducts and into the intestine, which leads to the stomach, where it helps metabolize (break down) fat.

The gallbladder is very likely to give you problems at some point. There is a period in our lives, usually in our forties, when the changes our body has experienced—either gaining weight or losing weight or undergoing a pregnancy—can affect the gallbladder. The location of the gallbladder is critical to understanding why it can cause problems: it sits on the right-hand side of our abdomen, just underneath the liver and next to the intestines and the pancreas. So it's anatomically predisposed to feel pressure from these other organs.

The most common disorder of the gallbladder and its bile ducts is gallstones, a condition otherwise known as *cholelithiasis*. It occurs when the liver begins secreting bile that contains too much cholesterol, which then crystallizes and forms stones in the gallbladder and the bile ducts. Stones can also form due to low levels of bile acids. Most gallstones are cholesterol stones.

How gallstones form is not well understood, but we assume that it has something to do with the way in which our diets alter the quantity or quality of bile we produce. The other possibility is that the gallbladder, since it not only stores but concentrates the bile, possibly removes too much water from the bile, causing some of its constituents to solidify and form gallstones.

More than 20 million Americans have gallstones, and approximately 1 million new cases are diagnosed each year. People over the age of sixty are more likely to develop gallstones than younger people, and women are twice as likely as men to develop them. But most people will walk around with gallstones all their lives and never even know they have them. Sometimes they're found by chance on X-rays.

When people do report gallbladder pain, it is usually because of gallstones or the inflammation the stones produce. When the gallbladder contracts—to excrete bile—we feel the pressure of the stones inside. So it's almost like holding a few marbles in one hand; when we squeeze our hand with the marbles, we feel the pressure and some tenderness. Gallbladder pain is usually felt on the right side of the abdomen, just underneath the rib cage, though sometimes it radiates to the back. It's easy to understand why people often complain of gallbladder pain after eating a fatty meal. It occurs because the body is demanding the excretion of bile to process the fatty foods, so we feel discomfort when the gallbladder, with the stones inside, contracts to excrete the bile.

The pain from a gallbladder problem may subside and then return in a cyclical pattern. This can happen when a stone becomes stuck in the duct system and obstructs the flow of bile, then after a few hours falls back into the gallbladder or passes out through the intestines. But sometimes the pain from the gallbladder can be acute; it's sudden, constant, and persistent. This is most likely to occur when a stone is jammed into a bile duct, creating a major obstruction, major pain, and a low-grade temperature, as well as nausea and vomiting. If the main bile duct gets obstructed significantly, you can have an acute buildup of bile, which then backs up into the liver and gets into your bloodstream; this causes a slight jaundice of the skin.

So what to do? If the problem is gallstones, you have to have them removed. The most common solution today is to operate and remove the gallbladder sack, stones, and all via minimally invasive surgery called a *laparoscopy,* in which a telescope-like instrument plucks out the gallbladder through the smallest possible incision. Conventional gallbladder removal, or *cholecystectomy,* is a major operation that requires a large incision in the abdomen, thus raising the risk of complications from infection and bleeding.

If a patient does not qualify for surgery, there are still several options available. There are medications, such as chenodeoxycholic, that can be taken orally in an effort to break up the stones; it is excreted to the bile and helps dissolve the gallstone. But these medications are not 100 percent effective, and when people stop taking the medication, the gallstones have a tendency to form again. Another possibility is a lithotripsy, in which external shock waves are used to bombard and shatter the stones; the same method is used to remove kidney stones, albeit usually with greater success than with gallstones. Still another approach involves injecting strong solutions directly into the gallbladder to dissolve the stones, especially cholesterol-based gallstones, but again, this technique is not totally successful.

By the way, in case you're wondering, there are no medical or health consequences from losing a gallbladder. The gallbladder is basically a receptacle. Even after it's removed, the bile is still going to be made by the liver, and it's still going to go down the tubes into the intestines and into the stomach. The only difference is that fat digestion may be a little less efficient because the bile has not been concentrated by the gallbladder, so if you have your gallbladder removed, you'll have to be particularly mindful of following a healthful diet.

Prostate Health (For Men Only)

I think there's a lot of confusion about what the prostate is. The prostate is one element of the male sex organs. About the size of a walnut, it surrounds the urethra, the tube that connects the bladder with the penis. The urethra carries not only the urine but also, during ejaculation, the semen, which is a combination of sperm and the fluid that the prostate adds to it.

The most common prostrate problem for men under fifty is *prostatitis,* which is simply an inflamed prostate; the symptoms are similar to those of a bladder infection: burning, frequent urination, and maybe some tenderness. The inflammation is often due to bacteria in the urine. Examining a urine sample under the microscope is usually sufficient for a diagnosis, and treatment is with antibiotics.

For men over fifty, the most common problem is an enlargement of the prostate, called benign prostatic hyperplasia, or BPH. One of the most common symptoms of BPH is difficulty urinating. Why? Because as the prostate enlarges, it squeezes the urethra, narrowing the orifice the urine passes through and making it more difficult to empty the bladder. Consequently, you might notice an urge to empty your bladder several times during the night. You might also have difficulty starting your urine stream. In some cases, you might even find a small amount of blood in the urine. But rest assured, just because you have BPH doesn't necessarily mean you have cancer, although sometimes the symptoms can be similar. The most serious consequence of an enlarged prostate is having a total occlusion of your urine, resulting in urine retention.

BPH can be diagnosed through a rectal exam; during this exam the doctor simply inserts a finger in the anus and feels through the rectal wall for any enlargement of the prostate. An ultrasound can also help diagnose an enlargement. Many doctors will do a PSA test, which looks for a prostate-specific antigen in the blood. But because PSA levels are elevated both in BPH and in prostate cancer, it's not a definitive test to differentiate one from the other. Other doctors might want to look specifically at the quality of the urine outflow by doing a urine-flow study and examining how much pressure it takes you to relieve your bladder, as well as looking inside the urethra for any sign of narrowing.

Mild cases of BPH are simply observed rather than treated. Many times the symptoms don't get worse; the prostate enlarges a bit yet doesn't really interfere with your daily life. More severe cases may be treated with medications that help relax the prostate and oftentimes actually shrink it. There are also surgical techniques that mostly involve shaving off some of the excess prostate tissue in order to significantly dilate the urethra. And there are nonsurgical procedures in which the excess prostate tissue is burned away using radio waves. Only in rare cases of BPH is it necessary to remove the entire prostate, that is, do a *prostatectomy.* One potential side effect of any kind of BPH treatment is the loss of sexual function, but most men regain their normal sexual function within a year or so.

The most severe threat to the prostate, of course, is not BPH but cancer. It is the most common form of cancer in American men after skin cancer, and it is particularly common in African American and Latino men. Few men show any symptoms of prostate cancer by their fifties. Prostate cancer tends to spread slowly in comparison with most other cancers; in fact, cell changes in the prostate may begin ten to thirty years before a tumor is large enough to cause any symptoms. As the cancer grows you might experience difficult urination, a burning pain, blood in the urine, pelvic pain, back pain, or painful ejaculation. By the age of eighty, more than half of American men have some cancer in their prostate, though most of the time these cancers never pose a serious health threat. Only 3 percent of those with prostate cancer actually die of the disease.

For prostate cancer, like all cancers, the fundamentals for a better outcome are early screening, early diagnosis, and, if necessary, treatment. Men should be aware that, as they get older, into their forties and fifties, there are symptoms they should look out for—changes in urination, burning, or lower back pain—that should prompt them to get a prostate physical. A doctor will give you a physical examination, a rectal exam, perhaps an ultrasound, and will test your PSA level. Remember that your PSA could be elevated because of benign disease *or* because of cancer. To distinguish between the two, a biopsy is usually required. In this procedure, a piece of the prostate is removed and sent to a lab for analysis.

The choice of treatment for prostate cancer depends on what stage it's in, whether it affects just part of the prostate or involves the whole prostate, and whether it has spread elsewhere in the body. If the cancer is growing slowly and not causing any problems, treatment may be delayed; this is usually the choice of older men who have other medical problems. The most common treatment is a type of surgery called *radical prostatectomy,* in which the surgeon takes out not only the prostate but most of the surrounding tissues and lymph nodes, too. Though side effects of the surgery once included impotence and incontinence, advances in the procedure have minimized these problems.

Another treatment option is radiation therapy, of which there are two kinds. One is an external approach in which a beam of radiation is applied to kill the cancer cells. The other involves implanting radioactive "seeds" in the prostate itself. It's important to know radiation therapy may cause impotence and rectal pain. If the prostate cancer is advanced, or is likely to recur, some men get hormonal therapy, which may cause hot flashes and a loss of sexual function and desire.

There is a lot of controversy regarding PSA testing, largely because the test can find cancers that would never grow or spread and don't need treatment. Nonetheless, it's the best test we have. Although a high PSA does not necessarily mean prostate cancer, the PSA is an excellent screening tool. If you have any of the symptoms, if there is a history of prostate cancer in your family, or if you have any other risk factors for developing cancer—like smoking, excessive alcohol use, or obesity—be sure to have your prostate examined now.

Ask Dr. Manny

SUPPLEMENTAL SOLUTIONS?

"Dr. Manny, I am fifty-three years old, and my father had prostate cancer when he was seventy-five. Is there anything I can take to reduce my risk of prostate cancer?"

There are several things you can try, but before taking any supplements, be sure to discuss them with your doctor. Many men with enlarged prostates have tried saw palmetto extract, a centuries-old Native American herbal remedy used for genital and urinary problems that has received enthusiastic support from many traditional physicians. Some studies suggest that green tea may also help prevent the spread of prostate cancer, and at least one study found that men who ate ten or more servings a week of tomatoes or tomato products had a reduced risk of prostate cancer. Vitamin E may also offer some protection, and many studies cite the importance of the antioxidant mineral selenium. But whether you can prevent or reduce the risk of prostate cancer by supplementing with selenium or eating more selenium-rich seafood, grains, and vegetables has not been firmly established by scientific studies.

Cancer of the Blood

Leukemia is a cancer of the bone marrow and the blood. The bone marrow, which is the soft material in the center of most bones, produces the red blood cells that carry oxygen to tissues throughout the body, the white blood cells that fight infection, and the platelets that help form blood clots and control bleeding. In leukemia, however, the bone marrow usually produces fewer normal white blood cells, thus increasing the risk of infection, as well as an overabundance of abnormal white blood cells. This results in a decline of red blood cells, which leads to anemia, and fewer platelets, which causes easy bruising and excessive bleeding.

There are about two hundred thousand people with leukemia in the United States today. Each year a little more than 10 percent of those people will die of the disease, and another thirty-five thousand new cases of leukemia will be diagnosed. Anyone can get leukemia at any age, but nine out of ten cases occur in adults, with a dramatic increase of cases in those over fifty years of age. (See also "Childhood Leukemia," page 22.) Men are only slightly more likely than women to get leukemia, and among ethic groups, the incidence of leukemia is highest among Caucasians and lowest among Alaskan natives.

Leukemia is not a single disease but is divided into four basic types. It's first categorized according to the cell type involved: either *myelogenous*—having to do with the bone marrow, or *lymphocytic*—having to do with the lymph cells. Then, it's determined whether it's *acute*—that is, rapidly progressing, or *chronic*—that is, slowly progressing. Nine out of ten cases of leukemia are of the chronic variety rather than acute. One-third of the cases of adult leukemia involve acute myelogenous leukemia (AML). Chronic lymphocytic leukemia (CLL) is responsible for somewhat less than one-third of the adult cases, and the remainder are about evenly split between chronic myelogenous leukemia (CML), acute lymphocytic leukemia (ALL), and all other unclassified forms of leukemia.

The symptoms of chronic leukemia, which are generally mild at first and gradually worsen, include easy bruising or bleeding, frequent infections, swollen lymph nodes, fatigue, headaches, weight loss, and fevers. These symptoms are not unique to leukemia, however, and may be the result of an infection or some other problem. Signs of acute leukemia include vomiting, confusion, loss of muscle control, and seizures. Leukemia can also affect the testicles, kidneys, lungs, and digestive tract.

A doctor can diagnose leukemia following a thorough physical exam—which checks for swelling of the lymph nodes, spleen, and liver—a blood test, and, if necessary, a biopsy. Leukemia causes a very high level of white blood cells and a low level of platelets. A biopsy, usually done in a hip bone, is the only sure way to test for leukemia in the bone marrow.

The cause of leukemia is not known, although a few cases can be explained by chronic exposure to benzene and other petrochemicals or to exposure to high doses of radiation. Other than avoiding such exposures, it is impossible to recommend any preventative measures, but the good news is that the treatment of leukemia aims to cure the disease and not simply treat the symptoms. Some patients may have chemotherapy; others will have biological therapy, radiation therapy, a bone marrow transplant, or perhaps even a combination of these treatments, depending on the type and extent of the disease.

Those with acute leukemia need to be treated immediately, while those with chronic leukemia are usually simply watched and left untreated until the symptoms worsen; when they finally are treated, however, they are rarely cured. Leukemia patients who survive five years or more after treatment are considered cured. The survival rate for leukemia varies from a high of 74 percent for chronic lymphocytic leukemia to a low of 20 percent for acute myelogenous leukemia in adults. The overall survival rate for leukemia now stands at about 50 percent, which is triple what it was a half century ago. New drugs and treatments for leukemia are under development and show great promise for the future.

A Cancer of the Defense System

Non-Hodgkin's lymphoma is the sixth most frequent type of cancer and one of the most rapidly increasing types of cancer in the United States, having more than doubled since the 1970s. There are more than fifty thousand cases of it diagnosed in the United States each year, with about twenty thousand people dying of the disease annually. You have a one-in-fifty chance of developing non-Hodgkin's lymphoma in your lifetime. There are more than twenty-nine types of non-Hodgkin's lymphomas, each one a little different from the next, but altogether they far outnumber the cases of Hodgkin's lymphoma, a separate and quite rare category of lymphatic cancers.

Non-Hodgkin's lymphoma is a particularly bad character because it affects the cells of the immune system, the very cells that should be protecting our bodies against disease. Specifically, it attacks the tissue of the lymph system, which is a part of our immune system. Your lymph nodes make and store *lymphocytes,* the white blood cells responsible for your body's defense against infections or other foreign invaders. The nodes are connected throughout the body by a series of tubes resembling blood vessels that carry a colorless fluid containing the lymphocytes from various parts of the body into the bloodstream. Because lymph tissue is found throughout the body, this cancer can begin in almost any part of the body and spread, either slowly or rapidly, to the liver and other organs.

For most patients, the cause of this cancer is unknown. Older white males are more likely to get non-Hodgkin's lymphoma than the rest of the population. Other risk factors include having an autoimmune disease, having a history of *H. priori* infection, being exposed to pesticides, and being on a diet high in meats and fat. There are many possible signs of non-Hodgkin's lymphoma, including fever, sweating, fatigue, and weight loss, though, of course, other conditions may cause these symptoms, too.

As with other cancers, the earlier you receive a diagnosis, the greater your chances for a successful treatment. Non-Hodgkin's lymphoma is usually treated by radiation therapy, chemotherapy, or through a "watchful-waiting" approach, which involves closely monitoring a patient's condition without giving any treatment until the symptoms appear to turn for the worse. New types of treatment for this disease are constantly being tested in clinical trials.

The Shaking Palsy

When we see people with tremors and a shuffling gait, we often assume they have Parkinson's disease. And more often than not, we'd be right. These symptoms occur when nerve cells in a part of the brain called the *substantia nigra* malfunction and fail to produce enough dopamine, a vital chemical that's needed for the coordinated movement of the body's muscles. Parkinson's causes a whole host of other motor impairments, including a stiff facial expression, stooped posture, muffled speech, and, in some cases, a total inability to move. The disease will also affect the individuals' mood and may result in depression, panic attacks, apathy, dementia, and a loss of sexual function. The precise symptoms exhibited and the progress of the disease itself varies greatly from individual to individual.

There are more cases of Parkinson's in the United States than in any other country in the world. One and a half million Americans currently have the disease, and another sixty thousand new cases are diagnosed each year. Parkinson's, which is the most common brain disorder after Alzheimer's, is rare in people under thirty; on average, symptoms first appear between fifty-five and sixty years of age. In any case, the risk of developing Parkinson's disease increases with age. It is also more common in people of European descent than in those of African ancestry, more common in rural than urban areas, and slightly more common in men than in women.

Most cases of Parkinson's have no known cause. That said, some cases of Parkinson's disease might be linked to genes, toxins, or head trauma. Studies indicate that those who have experienced a head injury are four times more likely to develop the disease than those who have never suffered such an injury. The rate jumps to eight times if a hospitalization was required for the head injury, and eleven times if the injury treated was regarded as serious. The antipsychotic medications used to treat schizophrenia and psychosis may induce the symptoms of Parkinson's disease. Although a number of genetic mutations causing Parkinson's disease have been discovered, and somebody who has Parkinson's disease is more likely to have relatives who also have the disease, a genetic link has not been established.

There is no simple test to confirm Parkinson's disease and no cure for the disease either. A physician may utilize blood tests and brain scans to rule out other conditions that have similar symptoms, but a diagnosis of Parkinson's can be reached only after a thorough examination of the individual. Treatment is geared toward easing the symptoms of the disease. Since most of the symptoms are caused by a lack of dopamine, the medicines given to Parkinson's patients attempt to replace or mimic the natural brain chemical in order to reduce the tremors and other symptoms associated with the disease. The most widely used drug for Parkinson's is levodopa, or L-dopa, but only a small percentage of the dopamine it produces actually affects the brain pathways that regulate movement; in addition, the drug tends to further reduce the body's own production of dopamine. Other drugs given to Parkinson's patients act by stimulating the dopamine receptors in the brain, but they, too, are only moderately effective because after a while the receptors become less sensitive, which results in an increase of the symptoms.

When medications fail, some Parkinson's patients will resort to surgery. But as with the medications, any surgery performed on Parkinson's patients can only help ease the symptoms. The most widely used surgery on these patients is deep brain stimulation, in which a battery-operated device called a *neurostimulator* is implanted in the brain to block the abnormal nerve signals that cause the tremors and other symptoms and electrically activate those areas of the brain that control movement. In the future, doctors hope to be able to implant cells that have been genetically engineered to produce dopamine (or stem cells that transform into dopamine-producing cells) into the brains of Parkinson's patients.

Therapy for Parkinson's often includes physical exercise as well as nutritional supplements. Physical exercise such as yoga, tai chi, and dance can help improve a patient's balance, mobility, and flexibility. Two nutritional supplements widely used by people with Parkinson's disease—L-tyrosine and ferrous iron—seem to relieve symptoms in a good number of patients. Parkinson's patients also commonly take large doses of vitamin C and vitamin E, as well as coenzyme Q10, to lessen the cell damage that occurs in the disease.

Parkinson patients run the risk of dying of aspiration pneumonia (see "Pneumonia," page 274). This usually occurs when swallowing difficulties lead to the inhalation of gastric acid, food, and digestive tract bacteria. Stiffness of their respiratory muscles may also increase their susceptibility to infection. Pope John Paul II, heavyweight champion Muhammad Ali, and actor Michael J. Fox are among the famous faces of Parkinson's disease.

Diabetes Again

The statistics for this disease are staggering. There are about 20 million Americans with Type 2 diabetes, a high sugar condition caused by poor nutrition, being obese, and a lack of exercise—factors that can all mostly be prevented. About two-thirds of the people with Type 2 diabetes have been diagnosed, which leaves about 6 million people walking around with undiagnosed diabetes. That's a huge number of people who have a very serious disease and don't know it. And that makes Type 2 diabetes, like hypertension, another silent killer.

Unlike Type 1 (see "Diabetes—Type 1," page 75), Type 2 diabetes is not a failure of the pancreas, but an inability to produce adequate amounts of insulin for a body that is out of control. On top of that, the insulin that is being produced is not acting the way it should, a situation called *insulin resistance* that occurs when the insulin can no longer stimulate the cells to process the sugar in the blood. This causes the sugar to build up in the blood, ultimately doing damage to the heart, eyes, and kidneys, and creating small-vessel disease. Type 2 diabetes is now an epidemic, and if not corrected in this generation, it will probably be responsible for most of the strokes, hypertension, and cardiovascular disease that we will encounter in our sixties and seventies. Type 2 diabetes is especially common among African Americans, Latinos, Native Americans, and certain Asian populations.

Most people develop Type 2 diabetes because they are overweight. Basically the human body does two things: it takes in calories, and it burns calories. When you consistently bring in more calories than you burn off, all those extra calories turn into fat. That fat first gets stored in the abdomen and the intestines, and then it begins to infiltrate the muscle mass of our body. And what you end up with looks very much like a marbleized piece of sirloin that you see at the butcher shop. That marbleization is one of the hallmarks of people with Type 2 diabetes. If you keep piling on the extra calories, the pancreas, whose function begins to slow down anyway with age, is no longer able to meet the demand for large quantities of insulin needed to metabolize all that sugar in the blood.

If you were to lose weight, a significant amount of weight, I mean, your Type 2 diabetes could disappear almost overnight. Yes, it's that simple. I, myself, was a diabetic. I had very elevated sugars. I was overweight, excessively stressed, and exercise-phobic. I had a very clear, black-and-white case of Type 2 diabetes. So I lost fifty pounds; I now exercise three times a week, and I've maintained that weight loss. Today I am no longer diabetic. If, like me, you have not had Type 2 diabetes for very long, and if you can overcome it by simple weight loss, you will end up with no permanent damage to your organs.

If you have any choice in the matter, diabetes is a road you *don't* want to go down. Just to give you an idea, here are a few numbers:

- Heart disease from diabetes accounts for 65 percent of deaths in diabetics.
- The risk of stroke is two to four times higher in diabetic patients than in nondiabetics.
- Seventy-three percent of adults with diabetes have hypertension.
- Diabetic retinopathy, which is damage to the vessels of the retina, creates about twenty-four thousand cases of blindness in America every year.
- Diabetes is the leading cause of kidney failure.
- One-third of people with diabetes have gum disease.
- About 10 percent of pregnant women who are diabetic may experience a spontaneous abortion or have children with major birth defects, including spina bifida.
- About eighty-two thousand people lost a foot or a leg last year because of diabetes.

The list of damage diabetes does to the body is virtually endless. If you are a diabetic, you must learn to prevent complications and stay ahead of the game. Being a diabetic is a full-time job, and there are several measures you will have to take to ensure you keep your health on track. You will constantly have to monitor your cardiovascular risks by monitoring your blood pressure and keeping it under control. You will have to watch your cholesterol levels. You will have to visit your ophthalmologist regularly to ensure you don't development retinopathy. You will need very comprehensive dental and foot care. But, most important, you will have to monitor and control your sugar levels. Several times a day you must take a glucose reading either by using Accu-Chek or doing a finger prick. You will look at your morning sugar and at your sugar two hours after you eat. For the most part you want your morning sugar to be less than 100 milligrams per deciliter, and you want your postdinner values, usually two hours after you eat, to be 120 and 130 milligrams per deciliter.

If your sugar is high, you will need either to inject yourself with insulin or to take an oral hypoglycemic. This kind of supply-and-demand treatment model may soon give way to more convenient methods, made possible by new research into diabetes. Devices are now being developed in which a sensor that continuously monitors your sugar levels triggers a tiny pump when your blood sugar is elevated to release small doses of insulin. Other new research is focusing on the possibility of transplanting the pancreatic cells, called *isolet cells,* into those who need them, in the hope of restimulating insulin production inside their body and minimizing the amount of insulin that needs to be injected. The hope is that this research will one day lead to a cure, whereby insulin will once again be naturally produced in the body. But as of right now, diabetes is not cured; it is treated.

Diabetes can be managed. Ultimately, if you're talking about juvenile diabetes and you start very early in the game by getting diagnosed and getting effective treatment, you can probably expect a normal life expectancy, but it's a very dedicated type of life. If you are now in your forties and you develop Type 2 diabetes, and you continue for a decade or more without any checks and balances, it's very unlikely that you'll make it into your late seventies or eighties. There's just not enough time in the pot. In other words, if you are forty years old, fifty or more pounds overweight, with high blood sugar levels and high cholesterol, and you don't exercise and you don't watch what you eat, you will without doubt see the effects ten to fifteen years from now. By the time you're in your sixties, you will most likely have hypertension, stroke, and cardiovascular disease. Don't go there.

Ask Dr. Manny

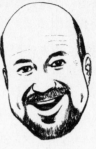

SWEET QUESTIONS

"I'm a fifty-five-year-old woman with two married daughters. We all have a sweet tooth in our family, and I'm worried that we might all become diabetic. Can people who eat a lot of sweets become diabetic?"

No. If you exercise and for the most part follow a balanced diet, you can like sweets and not become diabetic.

"Can people with diabetes eat sweets?"

If it's part of a healthy lifestyle involving a good diet and exercise, a diabetic can eat sweets.

"Can you catch diabetes from someone else?"

No, though some people think they can. Diabetes is probably largely a matter of genetics for Type 1 and lifestyle factors for Type 2.

"Are people with diabetes more likely to get colds or other illnesses?"

No. Your immune system is not compromised when you have diabetes. However, people with diabetes should get regular flu shots because any infection can interfere with blood-sugar management.

The Wonders of Plastic

Perception and aging have always traveled together, hand in hand. But aging isn't only about crow's-feet around the eyes, gray hair, comfortable shoes, and flannel pants. Aging is about the experiences that time brings. It's about coming full circle. I think it's a beautiful thing. There is nothing more elegant than seeing people appreciate their age and adapting their behavior to make the best of their life.

Many of us, however, are strongly motivated by perception—by how we want others to see us. The phrase "Keeping up with the Joneses" comes to mind. And it's not just about who has a greener lawn, or a bigger garage, or a fancier grill. Sometimes people treat their worldly possessions better than their health. I've seen grown men cry over a scratch on the hood of their car, yet they don't hesitate to light up a cigarette as they inspect the damage. The same holds true for some women; they can find time to shop, but God forbid they make time to get a mammogram.

I think many of us have lost sight of what is really important in life. It starts with those numbers we put on our age; then one day we get a kind of cosmic message: "Look at yourself . . . you're fifty!" That number may be a major kick in the gut for some, and so what do people do? Many reach for a quick fix: plastic surgery. Bigger breasts, defined calves, smaller thighs, Angelina Jolie–like lips, Nicole Kidman–like nose, hair plugs . . . you name it. But surgery is no small thing. Anything that involves going under the knife should not be taken lightly.

Of course, no one would argue the necessity of plastic surgery when women have reconstructive surgery after breast cancer; when individuals have rhinoplasty, a nose job, because the anatomy of their nose interferes with normal breathing; or when women who suffer severe back pain because of very large breasts get a breast reduction. These are all very good examples of reconstructive plastic surgery. But typically when we talk about plastic surgery, we're talking about cosmetic surgery, which is done to improve a person's appearance and self-esteem.

There is no doubt that these are boom times for cosmetic surgery. Inspired by all the body-

Plastic Surgery Myths

Do breast implants interfere with breast-feeding?

Do breast implants interfere with screening for breast cancer?

Do breast implants fix saggy breasts?

Is liposuction always better than a tummy tuck?

Is laser hair removal painless and permanent?

Can lasers remove stretch marks and cellulite?

No, no, no, no, no, no.

overhaul programs on television these days, more and more people are flocking to plastic surgeons for a little nip here, a little tuck there, to get rid of all those nagging "imperfections." Most of the increase in visits to plastic surgeons today involve minimally invasive procedures like Botox treatments to remove wrinkles and frown lines, collagen injections to enlarge lips and "erase" wrinkles, chemical peels to improve the appearance of the skin, and laser treatments to remove hair. But no one is ignoring the old standbys either: breast augmentations, eyelid surgeries, face-lifts, liposuctions, nose reshapings. And don't think for a minute that cosmetic surgery applies only to women, even though women tend to be the bigger users. Clearly men nowadays are also using cosmetic surgery to improve their looks and feel younger. For example, hair transplants, which involve transplanting hair from one part of the body to another, have been very popular with men who have premature baldness.

Liposuction is a technique that has benefited both men and women looking to remove excess fat from specific areas of their bodies. Liposuction reduces the number of fat cells in areas that are resistant to weight loss, but it is not an answer to obesity. It is not a cure-all for poor dietary habits and inactivity, and, in fact, when you remove large amounts of excess fat, significant metabolic changes occur in the body that could have serious effects on your health. The latest modification of liposuction is body sculpturing, in which fat is removed from one part of the body and injected into another part that you want to reshape, such as the chest and pectoral muscles, for instance.

Breast implants are the third most commonly performed type of cosmetic surgery in the United States. Though some women are concerned about silicone breast implants leading to breast cancer, no link has been established between the two. Nonetheless, the use of silicone has been discouraged in favor of saline breast implants. The implant is usually inserted directly into the breast itself, although it's also possible to place the implant on top of the chest muscle. Another approach is inserting the implant through the belly button, but it takes a great deal of skill to move the implant through the incision and all the way to the breast without creating a permanent tract of its passage through the body. Also popular with many women is the belly tuck, or tummy tuck, formally known as *abdominoplasty*. This is frequently done on women who, as a result of giving birth, have very lax abdominal muscles and very lax skin. Again, this is a major operation, in which all the excess skin and fat is removed and literally "tucked in."

The most popular type of plastic surgery is cosmetic surgery of the face. Face-lifts come in a variety of flavors, but all of them seek to pick up the slack in facial skin and reduce fine lines and wrinkling. Nowadays there are "drive-through" face-lifts, which are just mild cosmetic alterations done by placing and securing a thread in different parts of the face to hold the skin in a more rigid position. These fast, drive-through technologies have a temporary life span and do not yield the results that you would expect from face-lifts involving major surgery. Partial facial procedures include a *blepharoplasty*, which can remove the excess skin from the eyelids. This is quite commonly done because the skin of the eyelid is the thinnest skin on the face and is usually the first facial feature to show signs of aging. Suspension surgery of the neck and chin is done either by removing the excess skin or by placing sutures underneath the skin, in order to keep it tight. All these procedures are usually performed on an outpatient basis, and the typical complications involve blood loss, infection, and nerve damage, which are very rare, but the more detailed the facial reconstruction, the greater the chances of nerve damage.

If you are considering major plastic surgery for yourself, be sure to do it for the right reasons. What those right reasons are, I'll leave up to you, but think about it carefully. If you decide to go ahead with the surgery, be prepared to deal with the recovery phase, which can be quite an emotional roller coaster. The recovery, of course, is going to vary depending upon what kind of surgery you have. If you have a total face-lift, you're going to

What Happened to You?

Everyone has heard stories about plastic surgery. You want to avoid being one of those horror stories. Here are some tips to keep in mind when picking a plastic surgeon:

- Be sure the surgeon is board certified.
- Compare surgeons.
- Look at his or her credentials.
- Look at his or her previous work.
- Compare complication rates.
- Make sure the surgeon specializes in the part of the body that interests you.
- Make sure he or she operates in a well-accredited center.

be swollen and be black and blue, and the healing process will take months. You have to plan out how you're going to deal with your recovery. Will you be able to take some time off from work? Does the doctor operating on you have the resources to give you the follow-up care that you'll need?

More than 90 percent of individuals undergoing plastic surgery feel an overwhelming sense of improvement and a positive attitude toward their surgery. But 10 percent express regret afterward: "Why did I do this," they ask themselves? Some of these people will go through depression, which can be either transitory or quite damaging if not identified and treated effectively. But, thankfully, for the most part, plastic surgeries make those who go under the knife for the sake of appearance quite happy, even if only for a while.

Testing Continued

The medical tests that were infrequent or nonexistent during your first fifty years are now absolutely necessary, and in some cases even urgent, at this stage of your life. Waiting and hoping there is nothing wrong will not fix anything that needs repair. Remember that cancer risk increases with age. Beginning in this decade, an *annual* physical is recommended; it should include a digital rectal exam for precancerous growths (and the prostate in men) and a fecal blood test to check for blood in the stool and signs of colon cancer. Women should now have a mammogram every year. And both men and women should begin getting a colonoscopy every five years. Early screening means early detection; and early detection is when cancer is most treatable.

Picking the Fruit

For decades now, you've worked hard—and maybe lived hard. In the years to follow you'll have the opportunity to pick the fruit from the trees you planted—from social security, retirement plans, a paid-off mortgage on your house, perhaps, and—hopefully!—a healthy body and mind. The more you've thought ahead—either finance-wise, health-wise, or other-wise—the better off you will be.

Test Checklist for this Decade

☐	Physical exam (yearly)
☐	Colorectal cancer tests
☐	■ Fecal occult blood test (FOBT) (yearly)
☐	■ Colonoscopy (every five years)
☐	Prostate cancer screening (for men)
☐	Flu vaccine (yearly)
☐	Tetanus booster
☐	Gynecological exam (yearly)
☐	Dental cleaning (yearly)
☐	Bone density test
☐	Blood pressure check (every two years)
☐	Mammogram (every one to two years)
☐	Diabetes tests
☐	Skin check (every three months)
☐	Breast self-examination (monthly)
☐	Check BMI
☐	Cholesterol check (every five years)
☐	Blood sugar check (every three to five years)
☐	Vision check (every two years)
☐	Mental health screening (for depression, if needed)
☐	Hormone check (for women going through menopause)

We've Only Just Begun

7

(The Seventh Decade: Ages 60 to 69)

It's the decade of retirement.
Who me? Well, it is for most of us,
and eventually you'll have to decide:
What am I going to do now from nine to five?
Better have a hobby and make new friends.
Stay active, healthy, and wise.
Say, you haven't ignored your health
for threescore years, have you?
If you haven't no reason for tears,
it's time to enjoy your golden years.

Prostate
Flu Vaccine
Tetanus Bo
Gynecolog
Dental Cle
Bone Den
Blood Pre
Mammog
Skin Che
Breast S
Choleste
Blood S
Vision
Hearing
Mental
Pneum
Flu Va
Chest

If you've defined yourself by what you do in life, the seventh decade is one in which you will likely have to find a new definition. Retirement has a way of doing that to people. Of course, if you *are* your job, and can't see it any other way, you'll probably choose just to keep on doing it for as long as you can, and no one is going to talk you out of it. Frankly, that's just fine. The last thing you want to do is retire and be a couch potato. That's simply not a healthy thing to do. But if you have interests and activities other than those that have kept you employed for forty-odd years, this is your opportunity to begin really enjoying yourself—assuming you're in good health.

Don't forget, however, that at this stage of life your health depends increasingly on your social connections. It's a fact that people with a spouse, friends, and/or a pet have a tendency to live longer than those who don't have such a social support system. Funny how life is, isn't it? Turns out that we live not only for ourselves but also for others.

The other part of the health equation is how well you've been taking care of yourself all these decades past. How is your heart? Your lungs? Your colon? Your bones? Your hearing? Your vision? You need to take better care of your body now than at any time since your first decade of life. Remember that what was a minor problem in your thirties—like constipation—can be quite serious in your sixties.

Retire Late, Live Long?

Could it be that the later you retire, the longer you will live? It could be—at least up to a certain point. A study published in the *British Medical Journal* looked at the employees of Shell Oil who retired at fifty-five, sixty, and sixty-five. They found that people who retired at fifty-five were 89 percent more likely to die within the ten years after retirement than those who retired at sixty-five. They could not attribute this difference to sex, socioeconomic status, or the year the study took place. They did note, however, that the poorer health of some of the early retirees might have played a part in the results. The moral of this study? If you want to enjoy your golden years, you'd better stay active.

The Best Places to Live

A recent study conducted by Bankers Life and Casualty Company found the best U.S. cities for seniors to live in, regardless of whether they are retired or working, active or not, healthy or not. And it wasn't just based on the number of golf courses. Their criteria included housing, transportation, crime levels, environment, social opportunities, and health, which itself included factors such as physician-to-senior ratio, hospitals per capita, and availability of adult day care, assisted-living facilities, independent-living facilities, nursing homes, and senior meals. Here are their top fifty places:

1. Portland, OR
2. Seattle, WA
3. San Francisco, CA
4. Pittsburgh, PA
5. Milwaukee, WI
6. Philadelphia, PA
7. New York, NY
8. Boston, MA
9. Cincinnati, OH
10. Chicago, IL
11. Cleveland, OH
12. Salt Lake City, UT
13. Detroit, MI
14. New Orleans, LA
15. Indianapolis, IN
16. Kansas City, KS
17. Los Angeles, CA
18. Minneapolis-St. Paul, MN
19. Denver, CO
20. Greensboro-Winston, NC
21. St. Louis, MO
22. Nashville, TN
23. Providence, RI
24. Houston, TX
25. Washington, DC
26. Raleigh-Durham-Chapel Hill, NC
27. Austin, TX
28. Columbus, OH
29. San Antonio, TX
30. Orlando, FL
31. Tampa-St. Petersburg-Clearwater, FL
32. Norfolk-Virginia Beach-Newport News, VA
33. Newark, NJ
34. San Diego, CA
35. Phoenix, AZ
36. Atlanta, GA
37. San Jose, CA
38. Forth Worth-Arlington, TX
39. Baltimore, MD
40. Charlotte, NC
41. Las Vegas, NV
42. Fort Lauderdale, FL
43. Oakland, CA
44. Dallas, TX
45. Sacramento, CA
46. Riverside-San Bernardino, CA
47. Orange County, CA
48. Nassau-Suffolk, NY
49. Miami, FL
50. Passaic, NJ

If you haven't been taking care of yourself, this is the decade during which you're likely to have to pay the piper. Does the sound of that frighten you into finally taking care of yourself? I hope it does, because if you're extra careful, you can still avoid driving through some big potholes.

The Big Ticker (Heart Disease)

Clench your fist—that's about the size of your heart. Located in the center of your chest, the heart beats about one hundred thousand times a day, pumping five to six quarts of blood per minute. Once the blood receives oxygen from the lungs, the heart sends the blood from the aorta through the arteries and into the capillaries, which are smaller, thinner blood vessels. Then, once the capillaries have brought oxygen and nutrients to every cell in the body, the blood is redeposited into the veins, and from there it goes back to the heart for the cycle to begin again. So what we have here is a plumbing system essentially, a smart pump with different connecting parts that circulates blood throughout the body. The heart itself is made up of four chambers—the two up top are called the atria, the two on the bottom are called the ventricles—connected by a set of valves. And the whole system is set in motion, or beats, thanks to the electrical impulses sent out by a small bundle of specialized cells in the right atrium that act as the heart's natural pacemaker, causing the muscles of this organ to contract and relax.

Any malfunction of this blood pump is known as heart disease, of which one of the most common types is coronary artery disease. It is the number-one killer of both men and women in the United States. Half a million people die of it each year, and more than 12 million people have the disease. Coronary artery disease, also known as coronary heart disease, is a narrowing and obstruction of the coronary arteries, which are responsible for bringing oxygen and nutrients to the heart itself. As early as your teen years, fat deposits begin to develop in some of these arteries, and as time goes by, the fat deposits build up, ultimately creating an obstruction that begins to decrease the amount of blood to the heart and cause an inflammation as the artery tries to heal itself. Over time the fat deposits in the arteries begin to harden, and you begin to get deposits of small platelets that compound the obstruction. All of this can lead not only to a significant narrowing of the arteries, but to blood clots that may either obstruct the artery or get dislodged and create further obstructions elsewhere in the plumbing system.

One of the consequences of this narrowing or total obstruction of the coronary artery is *ischemia,* which occurs when there is an insufficient supply of oxygenated blood for the heart muscle. Any activity—eating, excitement, or changes in temperature—can make the problem worse. One of the most common symptoms of ischemia is *angina,* which is a discomfort, heaviness, pressure, numbness, or squeezing feeling in the chest. Sometimes it is mistaken for indigestion or heartburn. It is usually felt in the chest, but it can also migrate to the arms, especially the left shoulder. Other symptoms include shortness of breath, irregular heartbeats or palpitation, a very fast heartbeat, nausea, and sweating. If this ischemia is not corrected, if it lasts more than thirty minutes and does not get better, a heart attack may result. In a heart attack the heart muscle begins to fail, either through a very erratic electrical stimulation called an *arrhythmia* or by stopping altogether. It is important to recognize these symptoms because early intervention could save your life.

A doctor can tell you if you have coronary artery disease by discussing your symptoms, especially shortness of breath, taking your medical history, and looking at your risk factors, in particular, smoking, cholesterol, blood pressure, and sugar control. There are a host of diagnostic tests your doctor can do, such as an electrocardiogram (ECG or EKG); an exercise stress test; an ultrafast CAT scan, which looks for calcium deposits in your coronary artery; and cardiocatheterization, which can help determine the degree of obstruction of the artery.

If you are diagnosed with coronary artery disease, treatment is three-fold. The first has to do with lifestyle changes, like quitting smoking, starting to exercise, and keeping to a low-fat, low-sodium, low-cholesterol diet. The second aspect of treatment is medication, which may be needed to get your heart working more effectively. Other medication will be prescribed to reduce the cholesterol. The third aspect of treatment has to do with procedures to help improve the blood flow through the coronaries. One possibility is a balloon angioplasty, in which a small balloon-tipped catheter is inserted into the coronary arteries and then inflated to open up the clogged artery. Another possibility is placing a small, metal stent inside the artery to keep it open and improve blood flow. A heart bypass operation takes place when total replacement of the piece of the coronary that is obstructed becomes necessary.

Other types of cardiac disease have nothing to do with obstruction of the coronaries but with the way the electrical system of the heart works. Sometimes the specialized cells that electrically stimulate the heart become dysfunctional, and you can develop an arrhythmia, where the heart beats either too slowly, too quickly, or out of sync. These conditions can be diagnosed with an electrocardiogram, and sometimes medications alone can help to regulate the rhythm.

Another common problem is heart failure. This occurs when the heart can no longer effectively pump all the blood that it receives. Heart failure affects about 5 million Americans, and it's the leading cause of hospitalization of people older than sixty-five. Many times heart failure is due to prior damage caused by coronary artery disease, or by arrhythmias that have weakened the function of the heart. Ultimately, heart failure creates a backlog of pressure into the lungs, and people with heart failure tend to have difficulty breathing. Depending on the cause of the heart failure, different medications are available for treating it.

The valves of the heart are another source of heart problems. The valves can be damaged at birth or through infection. Abnormal or infected valves can interfere with normal blood flow and heart function and can lead to major cardiac disease. Surgery may be needed to replace the valves. Sometimes the lining of the heart may be infected, a condition called *pericarditis*. If this membrane is inflamed, the heart may not beat properly. Valve abnormalities, arrhythmias, and heart failure all have a common symptom—shortness of breath or difficulty catching your breath. If you have this problem, see a cardiologist to get the correct diagnosis and treatment.

The heart is a remarkable organ. It is the core of life, and its beat is central to your survival. Keeping it in prime working order is of paramount concern.

All for One and One for All

When we talk about heart attacks, we tend to describe them in a way that suggests there are different kinds of heart attacks. But those are just words to describe our experience of the same underlying disease.

Number one is the silent heart attack. Here you don't have major chest pain, you don't have shoulder pains, you may have a little palpitation, but you're not tired, you're not fatigued, and you're not dizzy. However, when you go in for a physical, the doctor finds that you have had a silent heart attack.

Number two is typical angina. This is the chest pressure that doesn't go away, and you have thirty minutes to get yourself to an emergency room.

Number three is the sudden heart attack. This occurs when you have a major, catastrophic obstruction in a main branch of the coronary artery, and a very large area of your heart is instantly void of any blood.

Even though the three heart attacks described here evolve differently, the underlying theme is the same—they all involve chronic coronary artery disease. In other words, you don't go around with a normal coronary artery one day and the next day develop a major clot. That's just not the way it works. The heart attack may present itself differently in different people, but the cause is the same no matter how we experience the critical moment.

A Heart Test for Venusians

What works for men, doesn't always work for women. We all know that, but medicine is just catching up to the fact.

The standard test for heart disease is known as an angiogram. In this test a dye is injected into the coronary arteries, which are then X-rayed to look for blockages. The test is very effective in detecting heart disease in men, but a new study has discovered that this test often misses the symptoms of heart disease in women. When the tests turn up nothing, women are given a clean bill of health, even though as many as 3 million women could be at risk with a buildup of fatty deposits that could ultimately interfere with blood flow to the heart and cause a heart attack.

Hidden heart disease may be a significant problem in women. It appears that one cause may be due to a phenomenon called *arterial remodeling*. This means that the artery dilates as plaque is deposited in the blood vessel so that, in the early stages of atherosclerosis or coronary artery disease, very little overall narrowing is seen on an angiogram. But late in the disease, the deposits may overwhelm the body's ability to compensate by remodeling, and severe narrowing or complete blockage can occur. If this happens, a sudden heart attack can result.

To diagnose heart disease in women, physicians will now have to use the new generation of CT scanners and magnetic resonance scanners, which can visualize the heart's blood vessels with ever-greater detail. In many cases, these tests can detect problems before a stress test or a conventional angiogram. Physicians should test for the presence of coronary artery disease in women who have risk factors for heart disease such as diabetes, hypertension, high cholesterol, a family history of heart disease or stroke, or nicotine use.

The moral of this story is: paying closer attention to the vast differences between men and women could save lives—in this case, women's lives.

Know These Symptoms (Stroke)

Your heart is not the only potential victim of cardiovascular disease. Your brain can be, too. Stroke is a type of cardiovascular disease that affects the arteries leading to and within the brain. A stroke occurs when the blood vessels that carry the oxygenated blood and nutrients to the brain are either blocked by a clot or break. This prevents the brain from getting the oxygen and nutrients it needs, and within minutes to a few hours brain cells begin to die. Every forty-five seconds someone in the United States has a stroke, and every three minutes someone dies of stroke. That's about seven hundred thousand strokes a year, of which about one hundred sixty thousand result in fatalities.

I can't stress enough how important it is to learn how to recognize the symptoms of stroke because it can save your life or the life of someone you know. The most characteristic symptom is a sudden numbness, weakness, or paralysis of the face, arm, or leg, usually on one side of the body. Other symptoms include loss of speech or trouble talking, blurry vision, double vision, decreased vision, dizziness, loss of balance and coordination, an out-of-the-blue bolt of pain, headache, vomiting, or altered consciousness and disorientation or memory loss. Usually these symptoms strike suddenly and without warning.

It is important to recognize the signs and symptoms of stroke because every minute counts when it comes to treating one. The longer a stroke goes untreated, the greater the damage and potential disability. So if you have any of the signs and symptoms of stroke, it is important to get help immediately.

Eighty percent of strokes are *ischemic,* which means they are caused by an obstruction from a blood clot or particle of cholesterol plaque that reduces the blood flow to the brain. The brain cells die within minutes of this happening. There are two types of ischemic stroke. *Thrombotic strokes* are caused by clots that originate in the arteries that supply the brain, like the neck arteries, or the arteries within the head itself. *Embolic strokes* originate from blood clots that form away from the heart but are swept up through the bloodstream and into the narrow arteries of the brain.

The other 20 percent of strokes are *hemorrhagic;* they occur when a blood vessel in the brain leaks or breaks. The most common risk factor for hemorrhagic stroke is uncontrolled hypertension, though it can also be caused by an anatomical weakness of the blood vessel itself, that is, an *aneurysm,* or by an abnormal connection of the arteries and veins in the brain.

There are several risk factors for stroke. People who have transitory ischemic attacks—a temporary halt to the flow of blood to the brain—have a ninefold increase of developing a full-blown stroke. At higher risk are those who have a family history of stroke, are older (the older we get, the greater the chance of stroke), and are African American, partly due to the high prevalence of high blood pressure and diabetes among the black community. Other factors include hypertension, high cholesterol, cigarette smoking, diabetes, obesity, cardiovascular disease, and high homocysteine levels. Homocysteine is an amino acid in the blood, and people with elevated homocysteine levels have a higher risk of stroke. Women taking birth control pills or hormone replacement therapy may also be at higher risk for stroke.

The good news is that there actually are some things you can do to avoid being a victim of stroke. Even though you cannot do anything about your race, your sex, your family history, or your age, since cardiovascular disease and stroke go hand in hand, you certainly can look at your risk factors for heart disease and hypertension and focus on early screening. Get your blood pressure checked; learn what your body mass index is; and check your cholesterol and glucose levels every two to five years. Exercise, manage your stress, limit your alcohol consumption, don't smoke, and stay away from foods with saturated fats. Take a vitamin B complex, like B_6, B_{12}, and folic acid, which are essential in helping to reduce the levels of homocysteines in the body. Don't take illicit drugs, like cocaine, which may trigger a stroke. People with risk factors for stroke should consider a brain-healthy diet that includes several servings daily of fruit and vegetables with nutrients rich in potassium, folate, and antioxidants. Eat foods high in soluble fiber, like oatmeal, to help reduce cholesterol, as well as foods rich in calcium and soy that help reduce your bad cholesterol and raise your good cholesterol. Foods rich in omega-3 fatty acids, which include, of course, plant oils, salmon and other cold-water fish like tuna, are also good weapons in the battle against stroke.

When it comes to the treatment of strokes, some hospitals have actually established special stroke emergency rooms that are manned by a multidisciplinary team well versed in their diagnosis and treatment. Whoever the doctor is, however, he or she must first determine the type of stroke and its location before treating it. A wide variety of diagnostic tests are available to the doctor, and they all fall into one of three categories:

imaging tests, which provide a better-than–X-ray picture of the brain; electrical tests, which record the impulses in the brain; and blood flow tests, which show any problem that may be causing changes in blood flow to the brain. Essentially, all emergency room doctors will attempt to improve and restore blood flow to the brain of a stroke victim. One way to do that is by injecting a clot-bursting drug, or *thrombolytic,* that helps dissolve the clot. Other techniques include performing a surgical procedure such as a *carotid endarterectomy,* in which the surgeon opens the carotid arteries and removes the plaque from them, or angioplasty, in which a balloon-tipped catheter dilates the arteries to improve the blood flow.

Once a stroke has been diagnosed and treated, most individuals end up taking preventive medicines to minimize the chances of recurrence. Some may receive antiplatelet drugs to make platelet cells in the blood less sticky and less likely to form a clot, or anticoagulants, which again prevent the blood from clotting. In cases of hemorrhagic stroke, where a blood vessel has ruptured, surgical intervention is needed to minimize further bleeding by clipping, cauterizing, or removing the clot and any vessel that is actively bleeding.

Stroke survivors must cope with a life-changing experience. They are often significantly disabled and, as a result, need a strong support system. Usually the support system is a team of rehabilitation doctors, which might include a psychiatrist, a dietitian, an occupational therapist, a physical therapist, a speech therapist, and social workers. A stroke victim has to deal with impaired movement, which has implications for walking, balancing, speaking, swallowing, and breathing; bladder and bowel dysfunction; and diminished sex drive—as well as all the emotional issues that result from those problems. A stroke victim's family is also profoundly affected because they now have to take part in caring for the individual (see "The Other Victims of Stroke," page 236). Stroke can change your life completely, so learn to recognize it and treat it urgently to minimize the terrible disabilities it can inflict on its victims.

The Other Victims of Stroke

The obvious result from a major stroke is devastating disability—such as speech impairment, weak hand and leg movement, and depression. But a stroke can also have an indirect effect on the health of the victim's family and friends.

Imagine a very strong and vibrant man who has never been sick, who has been a good husband and provider, who has been a great father. His family, and especially his wife of forty-five years, marveled at his strength. He was healthy and looking forward to a peaceful and blessed retirement. Then one day he suffered a major stroke, which left him unable to speak and walk. For the family, the confusion and shock were intense. How could this have happened?

This is not a fictional story. It happened in my family. When I first met my future father-in-law, I never imagined that one day his life would end up in such a way. However, this same scenario is played out over and over again in many families across the United States and around the world. All of a sudden, responsibilities that were the stroke victim's are now delegated to other members of the family, and in some cases the majority of the responsibilities falls on the spouse. From everyday things like shopping or paying bills to new responsibilities like making daily trips to the rehabilitation center; feeding, bathing, and keeping up with all the medications; and becoming a motivational guru.

All of this can have a tremendous impact on the caregiver's health. Suddenly, what was once an ordinary life becomes an extraordinary one burdened by the pressure and eased by the love for the ailing family member. We doctors sometimes forget about the families, and that's a big mistake. When dealing with stroke survivors, focusing on the family as a whole is always important. We must listen, support the changes that are needed, and monitor stress and the effect that it has on the people taking care of stroke survivors.

Family members take care of one another; they become the pillars of health care in the home and improve the outcome that any therapy in the hospital could bring. I remember the look of my mother-in-law as she dealt with her husband's disabilities, a look of love, duty, and compassion. But we must always make sure that, as we take care of others, we take care of ourselves. If you don't take care of your own health, you may very well end up being unable to take care of the person you love. So stay healthy. They don't say "in sickness and in health" for nothing.

Until Your Last Breath (Lung Cancer)

More than one hundred sixty thousand Americans die each year from lung cancer—more than breast, colon, and prostate cancers combined. Eight out of ten cases of lung cancer are due to smoking or an indirect exposure to tobacco smoke; the rest are a result of exposure to industrial chemicals such as asbestos, arsenic, and polycyclic hydrocarbons, or to natural radioactive gases like radon. Some have no known cause at all (see "A Fire Without Smoke," page 238). Some studies show that women who smoke have a higher incidence of lung cancer as compared to men, and women also die at a greater rate from lung cancer than men.

While it's clear that the longer you smoke, the greater your chances are of developing lung cancer, not all smokers develop lung cancer. This leads researchers to think that there may be an inherited component that influences whether or not smoking will cause lung cancer. The majority of lung cancer cases occur in people aged sixty and older, though by the time it's diagnosed at that age, the cancer has been under development for decades. The symptoms of lung cancer vary greatly, from difficulty breathing to coughing up of blood to a loss of appetite and weight loss to fatigue. But some lung cancers show no symptoms at all until they're very advanced, by which time it has usually spread to other parts of the body.

Lungs cancers are either of the small-cell type or the non-small-cell type. Small-cell lung cancer is responsible for 15 percent of all cases and is most prevalent among smokers. It's an aggressive cancer that spreads rapidly and responds best to chemotherapy. The other three types of lung cancer are of the non-small-cell variety. The most common of these is *adenocarcinoma,* which accounts for 40 percent of lung cancers, is most frequently found in women, and has been linked to low-tar cigarette smoking. *Squamous cell carcinoma* is slow-growing, causes 30 percent of lung cancers, and usually responds well to surgery. The third type, *large-*

A Fire Without Smoke

Everyone was saddened by the death of Dana Reeve in 2006. Who could not admire the way she stood by her husband Christopher "Superman" Reeve through the ordeal of his paralysis? Dana Reeve died of lung cancer at the age of forty-four. She had never smoked in her life. Many people wondered how this could possibly happen, believing that lung cancer occurs only in people who have been long-time smokers.

But people can get lung cancer even if they do not smoke. Ten to fifteen percent of people who develop lung cancer have never smoked, in fact. No one knows why, though the cause of the lung cancer in these individuals is thought to be a combination of genetic and environmental factors. Certainly, your risk of developing a nonsmoking-related lung cancer is greater if you have family members who have had lung cancer. And, notably, these nonsmoking-related lung cancers are more often found in women than in men. No one knows why.

cell carcinoma, is the least common type of lung cancer, responsible for only about 15 percent of the cases; surgery is the primary treatment for this type of lung cancer.

Many lung cancers are diagnosed at the time of an incidental chest X-ray. The lung cancer must usually be quite advanced to show up on an X-ray. Otherwise, the primary method for diagnosing lung cancer is through a *bronchoscopy,* which involves inserting a tube inside the windpipe all the way down to the lung chambers, where a doctor can either see or biopsy a specific tissue to make a diagnosis. Bones scans, CAT scans, and MRIs are used to determine the extent of the lung cancer—whether it has spread to other parts of the body, like the liver, the brain, or the bones.

Once lung cancer has been diagnosed, several treatment options are available, including surgery, chemotherapy, and radiation, depending upon the stage and type of the cancer. All of these treatments have their side effects, including fatigue, hair loss, diarrhea, nausea, vomiting, and anemia. Lung cancer survival depends on the cell type, the size of the tumor, the location of the tumor, and whether or not it has spread. More than half of all lung cancer patients die within one year of being diagnosed. Only about one in seven are still alive five years after diagnosis.

Currently there is no routine screening for lung cancer. But if lung cancer is so common, and if diagnosis usually occurs too late for treatments to make a significant difference, why is the medical community not more aggressive at screening? There is a national initiative to begin just such a screening program. The first step would involve screening people with risk factors for lung cancer. Is the person a smoker? Is there lung cancer in that person's family? The next step, still unresolved, involves the best screening tool for the job. Should it be a CAT scan? A bronschoscopy? Some other method? Which one is more sensitive? Which one is more cost-effective? Someday, I hope in the near future, we will have national screening for lung cancer. I think it will make a difference.

Gallbladder Cancer

Other than gallstones (see page 201), the other major problem that can occur with that bile-storage sack of ours is gallbladder cancer. It's common among Hispanics and some Native Americans, and more likely to occur in people who have had gallstones. About eight thousand new cases are diagnosed annually, with the highest incidence occurring in New Mexico, where gallbladder cancer makes up almost 10 percent of all cancers in that state. There are no symptoms in the early stages, though eventually you may experience abdominal pain, nausea, and vomiting. Gallbladder cancer rarely occurs before the age of sixty or seventy, and sometimes it's an incidental finding following a *cholecystectomy,* the operation in which the gallbladder is removed. Obesity is a risk factor in gallbladder cancer, and women get it more than twice as often as men, probably due to the stimulatory effect of the female hormone estrogen.

If you have symptoms, you can be tested for gallbladder cancer with a blood test. There is a specific tumor marker called CA19-9 that has been found in people who have bile duct cancers. If gallbladder cancer is suspected, a fine needle biopsy will remove a small bit of tissue so that a pathologist can determine if cancer is present or not.

Treatment depends on the cancer's location. If the cancer has not spread beyond the walls of the gallbladder, you can remove the whole gallbladder and thus remove the cancer. If the cancer has spread beyond the gallbladder and into the lymphatic tissues and surrounding organs like the stomach, the pancreas, and the intestines, treatment is more of a problem, and chemotherapy and radiation therapy are usually required after gallbladder removal.

Can you reduce your chances of getting gallbladder cancer, or bile duct cancer? Absolutely, by eating fruits and vegetables! That's the diet that will give you a healthy gallbladder. Why? Because that is what the gallbladder was designed for—processing the all-fruit-and-vegetable diet on which our ancestors once subsisted. It's also a good idea to maintain a healthy weight: if you need to lose weight, do it slowly, not more than a pound or two a week. You can also reduce your risk of gallbladder cancer by avoiding toxic chemicals such as dioxin, a by-product of plastics and chlorinated-pesticide manufacturing, and by not smoking. Cigarette smoke contains carcinogens that damage the DNA that regulate cell growth. And that is what cancer is: unregulated cell growth.

Weak Bones (Osteoporosis)

The word "osteoporosis" means porous bone. A porous bone is one that is less dense and, therefore, more fragile and more susceptible to fracture. Some 44 million Americans suffer from osteoporosis, making it a major public health concern. And it affects men as well as women. One out of every two women and one out of every four men over fifty will have an osteoporosis-related fracture of the hip, vertebrae, or wrist in their lifetime.

Some risk factors associated with the development of osteoporosis you can do nothing about. Gender, for example. Women tend to lose bone mass faster than men, and that has to do with the effects of the female hormones. Age is another factor we can do nothing about. The older we get, the more prone we are to bone loss. Body size is yet another factor. People who are small-framed and thin-boned have a greater tendency to develop osteoporosis. White or Asian women are in the highest risk categories; Hispanics and blacks are at a significantly lower risk. And if osteoporosis runs in your family, especially if your mother had it, then you are at risk for it as well.

There are some risk factors you can do something about, however, with the help of your doctor. These include abnormalities of the menstrual cycle—the absence of your period, known as *amenorrhea,* low estrogen levels, or premature menopause—that put you at higher risk for osteoporosis. The same is true for the man who has low levels of testosterone before his forties, or in conjunction with obesity. People with eating disorders, whether anorexia or bulimia, can have metabolic reasons for developing osteoporosis. A lifetime diet low in vitamin D and calcium also puts you at risk. Taking medication like steroids, anticonvulsants, or anticoagulation therapy for a long time can affect your bone density. Cigarette smoking, drinking too much alcohol, and leading a sedentary life all put you at risk for osteoporosis as well.

These risk factors suggest what you can do to help prevent osteoporosis. To begin with, you must incorporate calcium into your diet. There are many sources of calcium, of course, including milk products, leafy greens, broccoli, collard greens, spinach, sardines, and some other types of fish (see "Extra! Extra! Calcium," page 243). Most vitamin D is made through the skin from exposure to light, but as people get older vitamin D production decreases significantly; so people in their sixties and seventies should take vitamin D supplements. You also need to do weight-bearing exercises that strengthen your legs and your hips, in order to maintain a healthy vascular flow to the bones.

The symptoms of osteoporosis are silent; those with osteoporosis feel no pain. But some individuals, before they have any fractures, exhibit a loss in stature. If they have bone loss of their spine, of the vertebrae, you may see some bending of their back. This can create loss of height, spinal deformities, and maybe even some back pain. A doctor diagnoses the disease by doing a physical examination and perhaps a bone mineral density test, which you should have done every two or three years. This test is like an X-ray, and it can detect low bone density before a fracture occurs. It can predict chances of fracturing in the future by telling you how weak or strong the bone is. And it helps determine the rate of loss or monitors the effectiveness of treatment.

The treatment of osteoporosis involves good nutrition, a variety of vitamin and mineral supplements, and exercise. Even if somebody has osteoporosis, exercise is important. The only difference is that the exercises should be specifically designed for people with weak bones. People with osteoporosis should not perform any kind of strenuous, high-impact aerobics. Now that estrogen replacement therapy has gone out of favor, doctors are prescribing bisphosfinates such as Fosamax and Actonel instead; these medications help increase bone mass and reduce the incidence of spine, hip, and other fractures without the increased risk of breast cancer. The most common side effects of bisphosphonates are stomach upsets, and recent reports seem to link them to osteonecrosis of the jaw, in which the bone does not heal after dental work. So now dentists are very careful not to do major dental work in people who are taking these drugs. Another type of drug being prescribed for osteoporosis is raloxifene, a selective estrogen-receptor modulator. Raloxifene is also being used for the treatment of breast cancer. Several calcium-related hormones have been tried for the treatment of osteoporosis, too. One is calcitonin, which is a natural-occurring hormone involved in calcium regulation and bone metabolism. Another one is teriparatide, an injectable form of human parathyroid hormone, which regulates calcium metabolism; it also has been approved for postmenopausal women and men.

One of the things to take into consideration with people who have significant osteoporosis is fall prevention to avoid hip and spine fracture. If an individual has osteoporosis and has difficulty moving around, specific changes need to be made in their surroundings. This can involve installing bed guards and railings, as well as minimizing the use of stairs. Of course, you can use a cane; wear rubber-soled shoes for better traction; walk on grass rather than pavement; be especially careful walking outdoors in winter; and ensure that indoor rooms have no clutter, floors are not slippery, and rugs and carpets have skid-proof backing. In addition, don't walk with socks, stockings, or slippers, and make sure you use a rubber mat in the shower tub.

Ask Dr. Manny

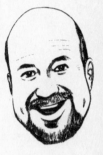

EXTRA! EXTRA! CALCIUM

"Dr. Manny, medical news can drive me crazy. One day we read that we should all be taking extra calcium. Then the next day we read that it won't do any good and may actually be harmful. What do I do?"

What you say is true. Medical news can be confusing. Often the more we study an issue, the more we learn about it, and sometimes what we learn contradicts something that we thought we knew about it earlier. For the past decade or so, doctors have recommended that women take calcium and vitamin D supplements to overcome the effects of osteoporosis and prevent broken bones. But a recent study of healthy women over fifty years old found no broad benefit from calcium and vitamin D supplements in this area. In fact, the study showed that an overconsumption of calcium could lead to an increase in kidney stones. However, it's important to realize that this study did support the original recommendation for one group of women: women over the age of sixty who took the extra calcium did show some improvements in bone density. They also showed that those who followed the calcium regimen closely for seven years were most likely to see a benefit. If you feel this report still raises more questions than answers for you, you should consult your physician about what is best for you. In the meantime, don't forget those other treatments to ensure healthy bones: doing weight-bearing exercise, stopping smoking, cutting down drinking, and, yes, eating a balanced diet rich in natural vitamins and minerals.

What Did You Say? (Hearing Loss)

Most hearing loss takes twenty-five to thirty years to occur. One in ten Americans suffer from hearing loss, including many relatively young people, but the prevalence of the problem increases to one out of three for people over sixty years of age. The aging process affects the entire hearing system. The eardrum loses its elasticity; the joints of the bones in the middle ear stiffen; and the number of sensory cells in the inner ear's cochlea, which contains nerve endings essential for hearing, declines. As a consequence, your ability to detect sounds at soft levels diminishes, as does your ability to understand conversations at normal volume.

Do You Suffer from Hearing Loss?

Hearing loss is often so gradual that most people who suffer from it are not even aware of the problem. Take the following self-test to determine whether or not you have a hearing loss problem.

1. Do you have to turn the volume up on the television or do you have a problem hearing on the telephone (cell phones excluded)?
2. Do you frequently have to ask others to repeat what they said?
3. Do you have difficulty understanding a conversation when in groups or in noisy situations?
4. Do you mumble or not speak clearly?
5. Do you have difficulty understanding women or young children?
6. Do you have trouble knowing where sounds are coming from?
7. Do you often misunderstand what others are saying and respond inappropriately?
8. Have others told you that you don't seem to hear them?
9. Do some sounds seem too loud?
10. Do you have ringing or other noises in your ears?

Scoring: If you answered yes to three or more questions, you could have a hearing problem and should have your hearing checked by a doctor.

Hearing loss is the third—behind arthritis and hypertension—most prevalent but treatable disabling condition among people in this age group. But only about one-quarter of those who could be helped with a hearing aid are actually using one. Why? The problem is really twofold. One, doctors are not very diligent about screening for hearing loss, with fewer than one-quarter of doctors doing so during a routine physical. And two, those who are affected by it are often unaware of their problem or are reluctant to seek help. (See "Do You Suffer from Hearing Loss?," page 244.)

Don't be. Whether unrecognized or unacknowledged, hearing loss often has a major impact on your psychological health. You may experience increased irritability, negativism, anger, fatigue, tension, stress, depression, social withdrawal, impaired memory, and reduced job performance. If you have hearing loss, you may require frequent repetition, have difficulty following conversations with two or more people, have difficulty hearing in noisy places like restaurants or malls, and typically have your radio and TV turned up very loud. You might also respond inappropriately in conversations, and you may complain of ringing in the ears (see "Ringing Ears," page 246).

There are several risk factors for hearing loss. A family history of hearing problems is a significant one. Certain medications can harm the hearing system. Chronic diseases like diabetes, heart disease, and thyroid problems, which are common conditions in this age group, can make hearing problematic. And, of course, people who have been exposed to loud sounds over a long period of time may suffer from hearing loss.

There are three types of hearing loss, each with its own cause, effects, and prognosis. *Conductive hearing loss* is caused by any condition that blocks the movement of sound through the middle ear. It results in a reduction of loudness and may be caused by blockage of earwax, a punctured eardrum, a birth defect, an ear infection, or heredity. The treatment of conductive hearing loss usually results in a complete improvement in hearing. *Sensorineural hearing loss* involves damage to the inner ear or auditory nerve caused by aging, congenital problems, viral or bacterial infections, an injury, exposure to loud noises, a fluid backup, heredity, or a benign tumor in the inner ear. It, too, produces a reduction in the intensity of sound, but it may also display itself as a loss of clarity, particularly of speech. This type of hearing loss is usually irreversible and permanent. A hearing aid is often an effective treatment for sensorineural hearing loss. The third type of hearing loss is a combination of conduction and sensorineural hearing loss because it affects both the middle ear and the inner ear; it's called *mixed hearing loss.*

A hearing examination conducted by an ear, nose, and throat doctor or an audiologist can pin down the cause of hearing loss so that the appropriate treatment can be administered. A buildup of earwax is simply . . . removed. Hearing loss due to ear infections require antibiotics. The treatment of underlying chronic disease like hypertension and diabe-

Ask Dr. Manny

RINGING EARS?

"Dr. Manny, one day my left ear suddenly started buzzing. It sounds as if I'm tuned in between two radio stations. Some days it's worse than others. What's wrong with me? Am I going crazy?"

Absolutely not. What you're experiencing is a very common hearing problem called tinnitus. It's basically a ringing, buzzing, or whistling sound in the ear that has no external source. Most of the time the origin of this ringing is unknown, but it's certainly very debilitating. Chronic tinnitus can be quite stressful psychologically and can be the cause of considerable nervous tension and fatigue. Treatments run the gamut from sedatives, antihistamines, and biofeedback techniques, to devices that mask the ringing by producing another sound. Though there is no cure for tinnitus, these techniques may produce some degree of relief from this extraordinarily troublesome problem. Make an appointment with an audiologist today to see what a hearing doctor can do to help you.

tes can have a direct improvement on hearing loss. About 10 percent of cases require surgery to repair a deformity or injury to the ear.

But most cases of hearing loss are treated with a hearing device of one kind or another. There are more than a thousand types and models of hearing aids. Though they differ in size, design, circuitry, and degree of amplification, they all have the standard components: a microphone for sound input, an amplifier to make the sound louder, a receiver to deliver the amplified sound into the ear, and batteries to power the device. If you need one, don't hesitate to get yourself fitted. It will do wonders for the quality of your life—and the lives of those around you.

I Say, Can You See? (Vision Problems)

Our primary means of relating to the world around us occurs through our vision. More than 80 percent of the information that we gather comes to us through our eyes, in fact. Consequently, the loss of vision can be particularly disturbing.

Our eyes—like all the other organs of our body—deteriorate with age. So just as kidney function begins to decrease when you're seventy, so your vision begins to diminish beginning in your forties and continues to do so

EYE FACTS

Diameter of average adult eyeball: 1 inch

Total surface area of the eye exposed: 1/6

Number of working parts in the eyeball: 1 million

Bits of information your eyes can process in one hour: 36,000

Distance your eyes can spot the light from a candle under good conditions: 14 miles

Number of images your eyes process in a lifetime: 24 million as you get older. That's just progressive and natural and can often be remedied with eyeglasses. But some problems are more serious.

Glaucoma

Two million Americans suffer from glaucoma, and half of them don't even know they have it, because most people don't have any symptoms initially. Glaucoma is associated with elevated pressure in the eye, or hypertension of the eyeball, and it's characterized by damage to the optic nerve, which can cause a loss of vision. About 5 to 10 million Americans have elevated eye pressure, which places them at risk for the disease, although glaucoma may progress even in the face of "normal" eye pressure. Late in the disease, visual disturbances occur, including a loss of peripheral vision.

Chronic glaucoma becomes more common with increasing age. It is uncommon in people under the age of forty, then increases until it affects 5 percent of those over sixty-five. African Americans are five times more susceptible to this disease than the average population.

Glaucoma is not a single disease but a myriad of diseases with one common factor—an injury to the optic nerve. The most common type is called primary *open-angle glaucoma;* others include *normal-pressure glaucoma*—a diabetes-related glaucoma—and *congenital glaucoma.* The treatment of glaucoma must begin by addressing any underlying disease such as diabetes first; and then, selecting a treatment depends on the underlying risk factors such as family history, old age, a history of heart attacks or strokes, diabetes, high blood pressure, nearsightedness, and migraine headaches. All treatments for glaucoma, whether topical or oral medications or a laser procedure, are designed to control the intraocular pressure and prevent optic nerve damage. People with glaucoma need to be continuously monitored by their ophthalmologist because this is a progressive disease; it's chronic but controllable, just like hypertension itself.

Dry-Eye Syndrome

A thin film, called a *tear film,* surrounds the eye. There are three layers to this film. The layer closest to the eye is a mucous layer, the middle layer is water, and the outer layer is oily. If there is a problem with any one of these layers, you may suffer one or more symptoms of dry eye, which includes irritation and burning, blurring of vision, and sensitivity to bright lights. About 60 million Americans suffer from dry-eye syndrome. It can occur at any time, but it becomes more common with age. The incidence of people with dry eyes increases from about seven in one hundred people in their fifties, to about fifteen out of one hundred people in their seventies, and it affects more women than men, particularly after menopause.

The causes of dry-eye syndrome are not perfectly clear, though there is essentially an imbalance of tear production and tear-volume drainage, one of the most common reasons for which is the normal aging process. Risk factors include other diseases, such as rheumatoid arthritis and lupus, as well as the use of medications like antihistamines. The diagnosis is based on the presence of dry spots on the cornea, and treatment almost always involves applying artificial tears in the eye on a regular basis, as often as four times a day. A humidifier in the bedroom might help also.

Cataracts

Just as a dirty lens on a camera will spoil your photos, so cataracts will spoil your vision with halos, glare, dim colors, and blurriness. A cataract is an opacity, or cloudiness, in the natural lens of the eye. It affects 20 million Americans and is the leading cause of blindness worldwide. The development of a cataract is related to aging, sunlight exposure, smoking, poor nutrition, eye injury, diseases such as diabetes and hypertension, and the use of certain medications, like steroids. About half of the population between the ages of sixty-five and seventy-five years have cataracts.

The treatment of choice for cataracts is surgery, and it's one of the most common and safest procedures in medicine today. In the three-step outpatient procedure, the surgeon makes a small incision in the eye, removes the cloudy lens with a surgical solution or ultrasound, and then implants the new artificial intraocular lens in the eye. You should experience little or no discomfort. The doctor will give you eyedrops to protect your eye against infection and help it heal. Because cataract surgery is so advanced today, doctors recommend that you get cataract surgery done early, rather than wait until your lenses are too occluded.

Eye Care

The decline in vision that comes with age is not totally inevitable. You can do things to help your eyes retain their youthfulness and flexibility. To maintain their optimum health, your eyes require specific vitamins, minerals, and antioxidants. If you are not getting your zinc from sunflower seeds, ricotta cheese, spinach, and other leafy vegetables; your selenium from shrimp, eggs, garlic, and Brazil nuts; your vitamin A from carrots, sweet potatoes, and winter squash; your vitamin C from citrus fruits and cantaloupe; and your vitamin E from peanuts, eggs, cucumbers, and corn oil, then by all means take them as supplements. You must also always protect your eyes from the sun's rays—wear proper sunglasses. Remember to release tension and stress by taking breaks from your work, especially from visually demanding tasks. Use adequate lighting when reading or watching TV. Wear protective eye gear when using power tools or playing sports. And always be alert for signs of vision problems such as frequent headaches, tired or burning eyes, blurred vision, and difficulty with either distance or close-up vision. If you suffer from any of these problems, see a doctor immediately.

Pancreatic Cancer

Behind the lower part of your stomach lies an organ called the pancreas. About six inches long, the pancreas produces digestive juices and enzymes that help break down your food so that it can be digested by the small intestine. It also contains small "islands" of cells that secrete the hormone insulin, which regulates the way your body metabolizes glucose. When cancer forms in the pancreas, it usually occurs either in the cells that produce the digestive enzymes or in the cells of the pancreatic duct that lead to the small intestine. These account for 95 percent of all pancreatic cancers.

Pancreatic cancer is the fifth leading cause of cancer deaths, following breast cancer, lung cancer, colon cancer, and prostate cancer. Each year about twenty-seven thousand people are diagnosed with pancreatic cancer, and about the same number die annually from this disease. Just 4 percent of those who are diagnosed with pancreatic cancer are expected to be alive five years later. This frightful prognosis is due to pancreatic cancer being very aggressive and difficult to diagnose early.

The risk of developing pancreatic cancer is low before the age of forty. Most people are diagnosed between their sixties and eighties. Unfortunately, symptoms usually don't occur until the disease has spread beyond the pancreas. Digestive problems, a loss of appetite, and unintentional weight loss are some of the initial signs. So is upper abdominal pain that radiates to your middle or upper back, although other conditions can certainly cause abdominal pain. About half the people with pancreatic cancer will develop jaundice, a yellowing of the skin and the whites of the eyes. In advanced stages, severe itching, nausea, and vomiting may occur. See your doctor if you recognize any of these symptoms.

The causes of most cases of pancreatic cancer are unknown. But it is believed that up to about 10 percent of the cases may result from a genetic predisposition. These occur when a person has a close relative who has had pancreatic cancer. You are also at increased risk if there have been breast, colon, or other cancers in your family. The majority of the cases of pancreatic cancer are thought to be related to environmental or lifestyle factors. Men are at a higher risk for pancreatic cancer than women; black men and women are more susceptible than other races and smokers are two to three times more likely to develop the disease than nonsmokers. People who have diabetes, are obese, eat a diet high in animal fat and low in fruits and vegetables, or work with petroleum compounds all have an increased risk as well.

At present there are no screening tests for the disease, but if your doctor suspects pancreatic cancer, a number of options are available to help image this organ, which is hidden behind your stomach and tucked inside a loop of your small intestine. A biopsy is the only way to make a definitive diagnosis, and a laparoscopy may be used to determine how far the cancer has spread.

Treatment for pancreatic cancer largely depends on how advanced the cancer is. The most common surgery for this cancer is the Whipple procedure, which involves removing not only the wide end of the pancreas but part of the small intestine, the gallbladder, the common bile duct, and perhaps a part of the stomach as well. Radiation treatment may precede or follow surgery, perhaps in combination with chemotherapy. If the cancer can't be treated surgically, radiation and chemotherapy are usually done in combination. New forms of therapy are being offered in clinical trials for pancreatic cancer, an option worth considering if the cancer is at an advanced stage. While there is no guarantee you'll benefit, if successful, the therapy you are offered could become the new standard of care for this ruinous disease.

Colon Cancer

There is no end to things that can go wrong with the body. And, of course, that includes the colon, the body's trash bin. The colon is that part of the digestive system where the waste material is stored until it is eventually ejected through the rectum and out the anus. The colon, also known as the large bowel or large intestine, is at risk for developing tumors, or growths, called *polyps*. These polyps are usually benign and not life-threatening. But if these overgrowths of colon tissue are not spotted and removed, they can become malignant. Over time, these cancer cells of the colon can break away and spread through the lymphatic system to other parts of the body such as the liver or lungs, where the new tumors can form. Colon or colorectal cancer is the third leading cause of cancer in males in the United States and the fourth in females.

A high-fat diet and a family history of the disease are risk factors for developing colon cancer. The association between diet and colon cancer is based on the fact that in countries with high-fat diets, like the United States, colon cancer is very prevalent, whereas countries with diets rich in vegetables and high fiber have a much lower rate of colon cancer. The association between family history and colon cancer is based on the fact that first-degree relatives of colon cancer patients have three times the risk of developing colon cancer as those whose relatives have never had colon cancer. So if your father, mother, or sibling has or had colon cancer, you run the risk of colon cancer as well. But most cases of colon cancer, a whopping 80 percent, are sporadic or spontaneous, with polyps the most likely culprit.

Colon cancer can be present for several years before symptoms develop. The symptoms of colon cancer are not specific, however, and resemble those seen in such noncancerous conditions as irritable bowel syndrome, ulcerative colitis or Crohn's disease, or peptic ulcer. These symptoms include fatigue, weakness, changes in bowel habits, narrowing stool, diarrhea or constipation, red or dark blood in stool, weight loss, abdominal pain, cramps, and bloating. Many times these symptoms vary according to where the tumor is located. If it's on the right side of the colon, where the colon is larger, the tumors can grow pretty large before you experience any symptoms. The left colon is a little narrower, so cancers of the left colon are more likely to create quicker obstructions of the bowel. Rectal bleeding may indicate that the tumor is located close to the anal orifice.

Several tests exist that can detect colon cancer. One is a lower GI series or a barium enema X-ray. A colonoscopy, in which the doctor inserts a long, flexible viewing tube into the rectum to inspect the inner lumen of the colon, can locate a polyp, biopsy it, or remove it entirely. The diagnosis is made by a pathologist, who examines the cells of the polyp. If colon cancer is diagnosed based on colonoscopy, either a chest X-ray or CAT scan of the lung, liver, and abdomen will be needed to see whether the cancer has spread or not. A blood test called CEA, or carcino-embryonic antigen, can detect a substance produced by colon cancer cells; CEA is usually elevated in patients with colon cancer, especially if the disease has spread. The treatment of colon cancer varies, depending on its location, the size of the tumor, and the extent of the disease. But most of the time it's treated by surgically removing a portion of the intestine followed by, sometimes, chemotherapy or radiation therapy.

The prevention of colon cancer mainly involves early detection and the removal of precancerous lesions like colon polyps. However, during your physicals, you should have a digital rectal exam and have your stool tested for blood. Then, beginning at age fifty, you should have a colonoscopy or similar procedure every three to five years. Any polyps found should be removed to eradicate the possibility of colon cancer. If you have a strong family history of colon cancer or ulcerative colitis, start the colonoscopies in your forties. There are now some genetic blood tests that can test for hereditary colon cancer syndromes.

One of the hallmarks of colon cancer is diet. By decreasing your fat intake and increasing your fiber and roughage, you can improve your intestinal health by preventing the carcinogens that might be in your stool from reacting with the inner lining of the intestine. Some reports claim benefits from the use of different supplements such as calcium, selenium, vitamins A, C, and E, as well as aspirin and some anti-inflammatory agents. But further studies are needed in order to recommend widespread use of these supplements or drugs to prevent colon cancer.

Keeping Up

Just because you're in your seventh decade doesn't give you the right to slack off. You have to keep your mind and body in shape with a little assist, here and there, now and then, if necessary.

Keep exercising. And if you don't already exercise, it's not too late to start now. At least thirty minutes, three or four times a week, is all you need. Walking is just fine. Walking ten thousand steps a day is a good way to help stay fit. Swimming is an excellent exercise, but at this age jogging and running are not the safest of physical activities. Exercise at this stage of life can help you manage your weight and improve your strength and flexibility, and it's good for your lungs, too. In fact, many professional athletes at sixty can perform better than sedentary men in their thirties. That's probably not your goal, but it's a good example of being able to do just about anything you want at any age with a willing mind and an able body.

And don't forget mental exercise either. Your brain needs exercise as much as your heart and lungs do. Read a good book. Play memory games like concentration. Do the daily crossword puzzle. Try sudoku. Challenge yourself.

Now that you are in your sixties, your immune system may need a little assistance to keep protecting you from outside invaders. It's time, in other words, for a few vaccinations. Be sure to get your flu shots in October or

November of each year; and, yes, it's still worth getting vaccinated if you've waited until winter. Late protection is better than no protection at all. It is also recommended that you get vaccinated against pneumonia and meningitis every five to ten years after age sixty-five. You want to do all you can to stay healthy and vigorous in order to continue the good life well into your seventies and beyond.

Test Checklist for this Decade

	Physical exam (yearly)
	Colorectal cancer tests
	■ Fecal occult blood test (FOBT) (every year)
	■ Colonoscopy (every five years)
	Prostate cancer screening (yearly)
	Flu vaccine (yearly)
	Tetanus booster
	Gynecological exam (every year)
	Dental cleaning (every year)
	Blood pressure check and thyroid function (yearly)
	Mammogram (every one to two years)
	Skin check (every three months)
	Breast self-examination (monthly)
	Cholesterol check (every five years)
	Blood sugar check (every three to five years)
	Vision test (every two years)
	Hearing test (every two years)
	Mental health screening (for depression, if needed)
	Pneumococcal and meningitis vaccine (at age sixty-five, every five to ten years)
	Flu vaccine (yearly)
	Chest X-ray (for smokers, or those with history of lung cancer)

The Beauty of Age

(The Eighth Decade and Beyond: Ages 70 to 100)

8

Congratulations are in order, for reaching the eighth decade. Luck certainly had something to do with it, but if you're healthy now, you're in it for the long haul. Now just remember this: Youth is a state of mind. You can be old at thirty, and young at seventy—and beyond.

We Are Lucky

We are lucky we get to age. Most other creatures on this Earth either die of starvation, predation, infectious disease, or a harsh environment long before they begin to show signs of aging. Only humans—and dogs, cats, and other pets we choose to protect—ever show signs of aging. And even that is a recent phenomenon. A century ago most people died of infectious disease before they reached a point at which the effects of aging really became very apparent.

In 1900, the average life expectancy was just forty-seven. Today, people can expect to live to 77.9 years and have a chance to show their age proudly (see "Life Expectancy," page 262). Infectious disease is no longer the major cause of death; now we mostly die of other causes, including the diseases of aging. The reasons why are rather obvious: we have a better food supply, better hygiene, and better medical care today than we did a century ago. Of course, that seventy-eight-year life expectancy hasn't stopped millions of people from living quite a bit longer than expected. In fact, there are 5.1 million people aged eight-five or older today in the United States. And more and more people are living past one hundred. Today there are about seventy-one thousand Americans who are one hundred years old or older. The census bureau predicts there will be one hundred fourteen thousand centenarians by 2010 and almost a quarter million of them by 2020. Most people don't want to live that long, however. Only a quarter of Americans want to live past one hundred, according to a recent poll. Most Americans say they would like to live to be eighty-seven years old.

But being old is one thing. Being old *and healthy* is another. While some people in their seventies and eighties are fit as a whistle, others are bedridden and suffering from serious disease, and yet others are somewhere in between. Eventually we will all reach the point when we can no longer keep up with the progressive damage to our bodies. But many of us manage to operate quite well past the warranty period.

The Bottle Is Still More Than Half Full!

I'm sure that people in their seventies would rather be thirty again—at least physically speaking. (No one wants to give up the wisdom that comes with age.) There is no question that a person who is seventy years old or more is a different animal from the thirty-year-old adult. There is an inevitable loss of body structure and function as we age. Our body reaches its peak performance at about age thirty and proceeds to go downhill from there. The following list assumes that the function of an average thirty-year-old man is 100 percent and shows the percent of function remaining in an average seventy-five-year-old man.

- Body weight: 88 percent
- Brain weight: 56 percent
- Blood supply to brain: 80 percent
- Output of heart at rest: 70 percent
- Kidney's blood filtering rate: 69 percent
- Number of taste buds: 36 percent

- Lung capacity: 56 percent
- Strength of handgrip: 55 percent
- Maximum oxygen uptake during exercise: 40 percent
- Velocity of nerve impulse: 90 percent

So your kidneys, your lungs, your blood vessels, and just about everything else functions at a different level when you are in your eighth decade from how it did four decades earlier. On top of that, by the time you get to be seventy or so, you're likely to have a little bit of hypertension, a little bit of diabetes, a little bit of coronary disease, a little bit of pulmonary disease, a little bit of a whole lot of diseases, in fact. No single one is enough to bring you to your knees—or worse. But it's very important that you maintain your vitality; otherwise, one or more of those little bits will eventually overwhelm you. So the good news is that if you are a healthy seventy-year-old, the bottle is still more than half full. The bad news is that you had better watch the other half of the bottle very carefully if you want to keep the sunset ahead of you rather than behind you.

Macular Degeneration

The eyes have it in our culture, so anything that threatens our vision can put a real damper on our lives. Though eye care should begin before the eighth decade of life, many eye troubles do occur at this age, including age-related macular degeneration, or AMD, for short. This devastating eye disease affects about a third of the Caucasian population age seventy-five and older. AMD is the leading cause of legal blindness among Caucasians, though it is, quite curiously, rather rare in other races.

Macular degeneration damages the center of the retina, the tissue that converts optical images to electrical impulses, which then travel to the brain via the optic nerve. Since this degenerative condition affects only the central vision, it leaves the peripheral vision intact, so it doesn't cause

The Heredity Factor

New scientific research suggests that genes may play a significant role in the development of macular degeneration. Scientists have identified two genes that appear to be strongly associated with a person's risk for developing AMD. Three out of four people with AMD carry variants of the Factor H and Factor B genes, as they are known; these genes are responsible for proteins that help regulate inflammation in the part of the immune system that attacks diseased and damaged cells. Scientists have also identified a gene on chromosome 10, called PLEKHA1, which is also associated with a person's risk of developing AMD. It, too, appears to be involved in the inflammation. Several other gene candidates are being studied to determine what role they might play in the development of this devastating eye disease. But to date there is no clinical way to test for this gene deficit or to know what type of inheritance pattern it has.

total (or "cane") blindness. To get an idea of what you are left with in terms of vision, hold your thumbs upright and close to the front of your eyes. That's all those with MD can see. And you can't see around the thumbs, as the impairment follows you around as you move your head. In short, it's pretty debilitating.

The exact cause of this disease is not known, but it is thought that the plaquelike metabolic deposits called *drusen*, which begin to form under the retina as we age, end up damaging the light-sensing cells, and as these die off, the vision in the center of our visual field begins to fade. There are actually two types of AMD, the "dry" and the "wet." The "dry" accounts for 90 percent of the cases and does not usually cause a total loss of reading vision. There is no treatment for "dry" AMD, but those who suffer from it need to be monitored carefully as the condition may deteriorate into "wet" AMD, which does cause blindness and occurs when tiny abnormal blood vessels develop under the retina, causing swelling or breaking and bleeding.

Treatment of "wet" AMD is still a work in progress. Laser therapies have been utilized to burn out these abnormal vessels, but not very successfully. Photodynamic therapy has been more successful in preventing further deterioration of vision. The procedure involves the intravenous injection of a photosensitizing dye, which accumulates in the abnormal new vessels; a red laser then destroys these new vessels. The treatment is expensive, however, requires access to a red laser, and must be repeated every few months. A new medication introduced recently, known as Macugen, has shown much promise. Basically, when it is injected into the eye, it interferes with the growth of these new blood vessels. The only problem is that the effects of the medication are temporary; it needs to be readministered every six weeks. And while it succeeds in preventing further vision loss, only a few people have reported an actual gain in their visual acuity.

While macular degeneration is a hot topic of conversation among those in their seventies, we tend to forget that there are some things we can do in our lifetime to prevent it.

First off, protect your eyes from UV rays by wearing sunglasses beginning at an early age. Nutrition also plays a significant role, and this is why I keep bringing up the issue of maintaining a healthful diet throughout your life. Studies show that people with the highest consumption of vegetables rich in carotenoids, like raw spinach, kale, and collard greens, have about half the risk of developing macular degeneration when they get older than those who did not follow such a diet (see "Masticate This," page 265). Smoking is another big risk factor for developing macular degeneration; in fact, smoking may actually *double* your risk of AMD. One final prevention tip: If you want to avoid macular degeneration, remember to maintain a normal blood pressure.

The Big Slowdown

Aging not only weakens our vision and hearing, but it diminishes our sense of taste, too, and this in turn influences what kinds of foods we choose to eat as we get older. Many seniors will seek out spicier foods, which may lead to gas and heartburn. Others will add salt to their foods, which can lead to water retention and higher blood pressure. Some older people seem to lose their taste for food entirely and simply forget to eat at all. Depression and loneliness can make this problem even worse. This is obviously a slippery slope, as poor eating habits will contribute to the ailments you suffer from as you get older.

The problem with getting older is that, while you need fewer calories than people in their thirties, you need the same amount of nutrients. That's not an easy trick to pull off by itself, but it's made all the more difficult by the fact that the aging process alters our ability to digest, absorb, metabolize, and utilize the nutrients in the foods we eat. Older folk may have poor dentures or fewer teeth, which can reduce their ability to chew foods that contain vital nutrients (see "Senior Smiles," page 268). Some seniors lose the ability to produce stomach acid, or produce an inadequate amount of it, which reduces their ability to properly digest proteins and interferes with the absorption of nutrients such as vitamin B_{12} and folic acid. Older people also produce less saliva, which contains digestive enzymes; this results in a decrease of enzyme activity in the gastrointestinal tract, which makes digesting certain foods all the more difficult. To make up for this, seniors should avoid eating processed and refined foods, which have reduced nutritional value to begin with, and focus on eating well-balanced, minimally processed, low-cholesterol, low-sugar, high-fiber meals from the major food groups—fruits; vegetables; bread and cereals; milk and cheeses; meat, poultry, and fish—and to take supplements to overcome any age-related problems with digestion and absorption.

Everything slows down a bit as we age, including our basal metabolic rate (BMR). This is the rate our body consumes energy while at rest. Our BMR drops by 2 percent for every decade beyond the twenties, so by the seventies our BMR will have dropped 10 percent. Add this decline to the natural reduction of activity that comes with old age, and you have a body that is burning significantly fewer calories. This means that you can't maintain your old eating habits without gaining weight. But you can compensate for this decline in the BMR with a regular exercise program, which can also help fight off the loss of lean muscle mass, which is another age-related problem. You want to keep your muscles fit, as muscle is more metabolically active than fat; in other words, the more lean muscle mass we have, the higher our metabolic rate will be.

The medications we take as we grow older can also affect our appetite and the way in which we absorb nutrients. But perhaps even more important, because our body has changed, the medicines we take as we age can actually affect us differently. Just as you wouldn't give an infant the same dose of a medicine you would give an adult, seniors should not be getting the same dose as an adult—for several reasons. First of all, our brain and nervous system become more sensitive to certain medicines as we get older. In addition, our liver becomes less efficient at breaking down medicines. And to top it off, our kidneys become less efficient at excreting them.

What this means, in short, is that as a senior you will need lower doses of medications than the normal adult dose to avoid overdosing and developing potential side effects. This holds true for everything from the over-the-counter Robitussin you take for a cough to the dose of penicillin your doctor prescribes for an infection. This doesn't mean that seniors should be taking children's doses of medications, however. Check with your primary care physician for proper dosages, which have much to do with how efficiently your kidney and liver are functioning.

Four out of five people age seventy-five or more take at least one medicine daily and 36 percent of them take four medicines or more. Multiple diseases mean multiple medicines, which increases the risk of interaction between medications and the chance of side effects. Make sure all your doctors know of all the medications you are taking, and be sure to take them correctly. Failing eyesight makes it difficult to read the small print on medicine bottles; arthritis makes it difficult to open up those childproof bottles; and failing memory makes it difficult even to remember what you should be taking when. It helps if you write down which medicines you should be taking, how often you should take them, and for how long. Keep a calendar with the medications and check off the day when you have taken them. To avoid mistakes, read the label of the medication you are taking, check the expiration date, and never take medicines in the dark. Don't be afraid to ask for help. You should also know what to do if you mistakenly miss a dose or take too much, and if any side effects are troubling you, talk to your doctor or pharmacist immediately.

And whether you are taking medications or not, remember to drink plenty of water. As we age, our

Senior Smiles

Other than children, those at highest risk for tooth decay are men and women sixty years old or more. The type and extent of tooth decay experienced by seniors is different from that which affects children. For older folk, decay often occurs around the edges of fillings and crowns, or on root surfaces of teeth that gum recession has exposed. In addition, missing teeth, sore gums, and poorly fitted dentures can make chewing difficult and contribute to digestive problems and nutritional deficiencies. So have your dentures properly fitted and your teeth checked regularly.

bodies don't always feel thirsty when we need water. Our bodies need six to ten eight-ounce glasses of water per day. So hoist a few glasses of that good-for-you crystal-clear liquid for your health. And this rule is valid no matter how old you are.

Alzheimer's

Here is a phrase you'll hear often among the seventy-plus gang: What good is being physically healthy if your brain is gone? One of the big fears as we age is dementia, the progressive decline—beyond what might be expected from normal aging—in cognitive function due to damage or disease in the brain. By the age of seventy only about 10 percent of this population suffers from significant memory loss problems, but by the age of eighty-five about half of the people suffer from some sort of dementia. And the most common cause of dementia is Alzheimer's disease.

Alzheimer's is an irreversible brain disorder without a cure that affects 4.5 million Americans. Put simply, it is a progressive degeneration of the brain's nerve cells, or neurons. For reasons unknown, these neurons break their connections with other neurons and ultimately die. Over time, this terrible affliction leads to loss of memory, impaired thinking and language skills, and personality changes.

What we know about Alzheimer's is that two types of unusual lesions clog the brains of those with the disease. There are sticky clumps of protein fragments and cellular material called *beta-amyloid plaques* that form outside and around the neurons, as well as twisted protein fibers called *neuro-fibrillary tangles* that build up inside the nerve cells. But even though we see these plaques and tangles in the postmortem brains of people with Alzheimer's, we don't know which come first. Scientists are unclear whether these structures cause the disease or whether they are a by-product of it. It's a chicken-or-the-egg problem.

Though we don't know what causes Alzheimer's, there is probably no single factor that explains why we get the disease. The greatest known risk factor is increasing age. The likelihood of developing Alzheimer's almost doubles every five years after age sixty-five, until the age of eighty-five, when the risk reaches nearly 50 percent. Family history is another risk factor, especially in families where individuals come down with the disease early in life. Those who have a parent or sibling with Alzheimer's are two to three times more likely to develop the disease than those who do not. Scientists have also found one gene that increases the risk of Alzheimer's, though having that gene does not guarantee an individual will develop the disease.

The changes in the brains of people with Alzheimer's probably begin ten to twenty years before any symptoms appear. At first, a person with Alzheimer's will get confused, tend to forget things, and be unable to re-solve simple math problems. As the disease progresses, the symptoms become more noticeable. People in the middle stages of Alzheimer's will forget to do the simple things in life like taking a bath, combing their hair, cleaning their teeth. They will fail to recognize familiar places, their sur-roundings, and their families. As they lose touch with what is going on, they become frightened, anxious, and aggressive. Eventually most of these patients need complete care. The average time from onset of the symptoms to total disruption of daily function is about eight to ten years. Some people manage to live with Alzheimer's for up to twenty years.

The only way to definitively diagnose Alzheimer's is postmortem, through an autopsy. Because there are so many other diseases that can mimic this illness, it's very important when Alzheimer's is suspected to find a doctor who is able to distinguish between Alzheimer's and some other forms of dementia. The right doctor will know how to use a variety of neurological imaging devices to look for and pinpoint the plaques that are characteristic of Alzheimer's and measure the progression of disease.

At present there's no treatment whatsoever for Alzheimer's. Drugs like Cognex or Aricept may be given in the early to early middle stages of the disease to alleviate the symptoms and reduce the sufferer's agitation, lack of sleep, and depression. At the very least, the drugs make the scenario easier to deal with for the caregiver. Since the plaques may be creating an inflammatory response in the surrounding brain tissue, nonsteroidal anti-inflammatory medicines such as ibuprofen have been shown to help slow the progress of Alzheimer's disease. Some reports suggest that the use of antioxidants like vitamin E and vitamin C can also slow the disease, while ginkgo biloba supplements seem to improve cognitive functioning, but there's really no evidence that such vitamins and supplements are truly effective. Since the way the brain degenerates in Alzheimer's disease somewhat resembles the way in which the brain is affected in diabetes, some treatments for Alzheimer's patients concentrate on improving their diet, and the recommended diet is one that's rich in vegetables and low in fat.

The problem with Alzheimer's, aside from being one of the most difficult diseases that anybody can have, is that it not only affects the individual but, as with stroke patients, it affects the physical and mental health of the victim's entire family. Families and spouses end up having to provide day-to-day care for these people, and it's often very difficult to do so. The Alzheimer's Association, with its multiple chapters around the country, does the best it can to provide support and information to families with an Alzheimer's sufferer.

Ovarian Cancer

Ovarian cancer is another silent killer. Often in ovarian cancer there are no symptoms until the cancer has spread well beyond the ovaries. That's one of the saddest things about a diagnosis of ovarian cancer; it's often too late to save the woman's life. Ovarian tissue is very complex, with more than thirty different types of cells, meaning that about thirty different types of ovarian cancer can develop, each with its own aggressiveness, malignancy, and occurrence.

All women are at risk for developing ovarian cancer, though the biological events that lead to it are unknown. As in most forms of cancer, not only does risk increase with age, but a family history of the disease appears to play a role as well. A woman has as much as a 50 percent risk of getting ovarian cancer if two or more first-degree relatives—mother, sister, daughter—or second-degree relatives—grandmother, aunt—have had the cancer themselves. Family inheritance can occur in one of three ways. Rare is the *site-specific ovarian cancer syndrome,* in which multiple family members have been affected by ovarian cancer only. More common is *breast/ovarian cancer syndrome,* in which the relatives have had breast and/or ovarian cancers. The third type, called *lynch syndrome II,* applies to women with either female or male relatives with nonpolyp colon cancer and other cancers of the kidneys, pancreas, and other sites.

There also seems to be a relationship between the number of menstrual cycles a woman has in her life and her risk of ovarian cancer. If you began your menses before the age of twelve or if you experienced menopause after the age of fifty, then you are at increased risk of ovarian cancer. A woman who has never been pregnant is at greater risk than one who has had children; in fact, multiple pregnancies seem to have a protective effect, as do birth control pills. On the other hand, fertility treatments for in vitro fertilization, which hyperstimulate ovaries to produce more eggs, are another common risk factor for ovarian cancer.

Other risk factors include diets high in animal fats, which have been statistically linked to higher rates of ovarian cancer. In a country like Japan, where diets are generally low in fat, ovarian cancer rates are low. In conjunction with this, one of the hallmarks of this type of cancer is an enlarged abdominal girth (see "Which Fruit Are You?," page 232). Talcum powder has also been suspected of increasing the risk for ovarian cancer. Women used to apply talcum powder on their genitals or on their sanitary napkins, and at one time talc was contaminated with asbestos, a known cancer-causing substance. Talc is now asbestos-free, but suspicions of its carcinogenicity remain.

The early symptoms of ovarian cancer are often vague, making this disease difficult to detect. There may be some abdominal or pelvic discomfort, pain during intercourse, bloating that is not relieved by over-the-counter antacids, changes in bowel function (either constipation or diarrhea), maybe nausea, vomiting, or unusual vaginal bleeding. Most often these symptoms do not indicate ovarian cancer, however; they are not distinctive. That's why three-quarters of ovarian cancers have spread to the abdomen by the time they are detected, and most of the women who have come down with this cancer die within five years.

If detected early, ovarian cancer has a 90 percent cure rate. Unfortunately, three out of four women are diagnosed in later stages, when survival drops to about 30 percent. So why don't we pick up more cases of ovarian cancer early on? The problem is that we don't have a good screening tool, or at least there has been no consensus on the best screening tool for ovarian cancer. A blood test can pick up a tumor marker called CA 125, but there are a lot of things besides ovarian cancer that can alter these tumor markers. Ultrasounds, which are based on the fact that solids reflect sounds waves, can show tumors in the ovaries, but they cannot distinguish between cancerous masses and those caused by benign disease. Since there is no national screening program, ovarian cancer is usually caught early on only when it is detected during a woman's regular gynecological examination. The doctor will palpate the ovaries during a pelvic and rectal exam for the presence of ovarian cysts or tumors. If any abnormality is found, especially in a woman over fifty, the doctor will follow up with an X-ray, an ultrasound, a CAT scan, and, if necessary, a laproscopy, a surgical procedure that employs a slender, tubular instrument to biopsy the suspected ovarian mass.

A hysterectomy most often follows the diagnosis of ovarian cancer. Because this cancer is what is known as a *surface spreader*, if the lesion is confined to the ovary, removing the ovary and the surrounding tissues is usually effective and sufficient. If, on the other hand, there is massive spread of the cancer, surgeons will perform what's called a *de-bulking pro-*

cedure, which attempts to remove as much of the cancer as possible, followed by chemotherapy and radiation therapy to wipe out any remaining cancer cells. In short, the survival of an ovarian cancer patient is based on the type of ovarian cancer, whether it has spread beyond the ovary, and how successful the doctor has been in removing it all.

Pneumonia

The very young and the very old are alike in many ways in terms of health, and you'll hear the comparison often. That, in fact, is the case with pneumonia. The two groups of people most susceptible to pneumonia are the very young and adults over the age of sixty-five. What could these two groups possibly have in common? Answer: An immune system that is not up to the task. In short, pneumonia is the scourge of a weakened immune system. In the very young, the immune system is not fully developed, and in people over sixty-five the immune system is beginning to fail. Why? Because this older population has more chronic illness, more history of cardiovascular disease, more history of emphysema, more history of diabetes, and is more likely to have been treated with chemotherapy for some sort of cancer than any other segment of the population.

Pneumonia is an inflammation of the lungs that's usually caused by an infection from bacteria, viruses, funguses, or anything else that can grow in the lungs. There are about fifty different types of pneumonia, but the most common ones are bacterial pneumonias, which usually produce chills, high fever, sweating, chest pain when you breathe, and coughing with thick green or yellow mucus. Viral pneumonias are more frequent in the wintertime and are very common among people with a long history of cardiovascular lung disease like emphysema. A viral pneumonia will start with a nonproductive cough (one without sputum or phlegm), followed by fever, muscle ache, fatigue, and difficulties breathing.

Pneumonia is not a contagious disease, so you can't catch it from somebody else, but there are many places to pick up the bacteria, viruses, and fungi that can cause pneumonia. You will be exposed to some of them in the course of your everyday life; these are called community-acquired pneumonias. Elderly people on a ventilator or in the intensive care unit of a hospital often get what's called hospital-acquired pneumonia, because of all the bugs that are prevalent in hospitals. Some people, as they get older, can lose their gag reflex and get aspiration pneumonia; that's when some of the contents of the stomach is regurgitated into the back of their throat and falls into their lungs.

Pneumonia can be life-threatening. If you're sixty-five or older, and you think you have pneumonia, the earlier you see a doctor, the better. If you are coughing and are experiencing a shortness of breath along with an unexplained fever of 102, seek attention immediately. Because if you have pneumonia *and* you're in those upper decades of life *and* you have other medical problems, you could be dead in twenty-four hours.

A doctor can diagnosis pneumonia by doing a chest X-ray, by checking for bacteria in your bloodstream or in your sputum, or by finding a fluid accumulation in the lungs with a *bronchoscope,* which is a thin viewing instrument that allows the doctor to examine your airways. If it's bacterial pneumonia, you'll be treated with aggressive antibiotics, while viral pneumonias get antiviral medications. Special medications are available if the pneumonia is due to a fungus like mycoplasma. Plenty of rest and fluids are always recommended for pneumonia. Most severe pneumonias in older patients are usually treated in the hospital. Pneumonia is not something you want to fool around with; it needs to be treated very aggressively.

The best way to prevent pneumonia is to keep your immune system strong. One way to do this is by getting your annual flu shot, which everyone should get but especially those who are over sixty-five. There's also a pneumonia vaccine that older folks should get, especially those whose immune systems are compromised by some other disease. The other hallmarks of prevention have to do with a healthy lifestyle—don't smoke, eat a balanced diet, and get proper rest. Oh, and wash your hands regularly, too. That's a good rule for everyone, but especially so for the very young and for senior citizens.

Home Safety Tips

Every year more than 1 million people over the age of sixty-five are treated in a hospital for injuries related to the things they use at home every day. Take a few moments to spot and correct any safety hazards in your home.

- Do your rugs and carpets have nonskid backing?
- Are your electrical cords out of the way of traffic?
- Do you have a nonslip mat in the shower or bathtub?
- Are your countertop appliances unplugged when not in use?
- Do you have fresh batteries in your smoke detectors and carbon monoxide alarms?
- Are your lightbulbs the correct type and wattage? (If you are unsure, use 60 watts or less to prevent accidental fires.)
- Can you easily reach a lamp or light switch from your bed for nighttime safety?
- Do you have a battery-powered flashlight easily available at all times?
- Are your radios, TV, telephones, and other appliances kept away from sinks, tubs, and showers?

Test Checklist for this Decade

☐	Pneumococcal vaccine
☐	Flu vaccine (yearly)
☐	Dental cleaning (yearly)
☐	Skin check (every three months)
☐	Blood pressure and thyroid function check (yearly)
☐	Cholesterol check (every five years)
☐	Blood sugar check (every three to five years)
☐	Colorectal cancer tests
	■ Fecal occult blood test (FOBT) (every year)
	■ Colonoscopy (every five years)
☐	Prostate cancer screening (yearly)
☐	Breast self-examination (monthly)
☐	Gynecological exam (every year)
☐	Mental health screening (for depression, if needed)

Living Long

Beyond the litany you know well by now—not smoking, eating well, and exercising regularly—there are a few other lifestyle choices to keep in mind if you care to stretch out your years as long as possible. First of all, have a positive attitude. Researchers have found that people who are optimistic decreased their risk of early death by half over their more pessimistic counterparts. Let your mind rule your body, not the other way around. Think positively.

Some researchers have found that being conscientious may also be related to living long, and by that they mean more than just looking both ways before crossing the street, though that will certainly increase your chances of a longer life. It seems that those who rate low on a conscientiousness scale tend to die sooner than those who rate high, perhaps because the latter tend to react constructively to emotional and social situations and are more likely to create a healthy work and living environment for themselves. So do what you think is "right," and do it with care.

Having a pet can also add years to your life, apparently. In one study, the survival rates of heart attack victims who had a pet were 38 percent higher than those who did not have an animal companion. There's no hocus-pocus needed to explain why this could happen. To begin, contact with a familiar animal seems to trigger a relaxation response, reducing our level of stress. Furthermore, pets have a knack for getting people off their duff and moving. How many people would never get any exercise if it weren't for their dogs?

One more thing. Taking care of other people—not just pets—also has a positive effect on life span. Have you noticed how many old folk die soon after their spouse has passed away? There seems to be something about being needed that helps us hang in there a little longer. So take care of someone who needs your help; it will be good for them and for you, too.

I wish to correct one misconception before bringing this book to a close. Back in 1965, rock star Pete Townshend of the Who wrote the lyric, "I hope I die before I get old." But it turns out that Pete, like so many of us, was operating on the mistaken belief that the happiest days of our lives occur when we're young. A recent study conducted at the University of Michigan suggests that, quite to the contrary, people tend to become happier over time. It seems that people, as they age, get better at managing life's ups and downs, and the result is that they become happier, even though their circumstances, such as their health, decline. I think that what Pete should have written instead is rather obvious: "I hope I get old before I die."

May you all arrive healthy and happy into your sunset years . . . and keep right on going.

The Master Checklist of Tests and Vaccinations

The Tests	Why You Need It	When and How Often	What to Expect	What the Results Mean
Amniocentesis	For pregnant mothers, to check for genetic defects in the fetus, if you are over thirty-five, if you have an abnormal "triple screen" blood test or first trimester screen, or if there is a history of birth defects in the family. Or to check for infections or on lung development.	To test for fetal abnormalities, anytime between the 14th and 20th weeks of pregnancy. To check on fetal lung development, late in the third trimester.	A hollow needle several inches long is inserted through your abdominal muscle and through the wall of the uterus to collect a sample of the fluid that surrounds the fetus. You may experience a stinging sensation. The baby's and mother's hearts are checked at the beginning and at end of the procedure, which takes about half an hour.	Tests of fetal cells found in this fluid can reveal the presence of Down's syndrome or other chromosome problems. Also shows whether the baby's lungs are mature enough for survival.
APGAR Test	To quickly check the overall condition of the newborn within minutes of birth.	One minute after birth and again at five minutes after birth.	The doctor will score how well the baby is doing on five measures: skin tone, respiration, heart rate, muscle tone, and reflexes.	A score of 7 or more on a scale of 10 indicates that the baby is in good health. A lower score simply means that the baby needs immediate care, such as a suctioning of the airways or a little oxygen to help with breathing. The

The Tests	Why You Need It	When and How Often	What to Expect	What the Results Mean
				APGAR test is not a measure of the baby's long-term health
Blood Pressure Check	To find out if you have high blood pressure, or hypertension, which is known as the "silent killer" because the condition rarely displays symptoms.	Check occasionally beginning at age two. Then every two years beginning at twenty-one.	The doctor taking your blood pressure will put a cuff around the top of your arm, pump up the cuff, then listen for the flow of blood through a stethoscope placed in the hollow of your elbow as the mercury column drops in the instrument called a sphygmomanometer. It's quick and painless.	Normal: less than 120/80; Prehypertension: 120–139/80–89; High Stage 1: 140–159/90–99; High Stage 2: 160 or higher/ 100 or higher. If blood pressure is high, the doctor may recommend a new diet, an exercise program, life style changes, as well as possible medication.
Blood Sugar Test (Glucose Screening)	To check for diabetes or to monitor the treatment of diabetes. A blood glucose test measures the amount of a type of sugar, called glucose, in your blood.	When pregnant, and every three to five years beginning in the forties for both men and women. Earlier if you are overweight or have a family history of diabetes.	You will be asked to drink a sugary liquid, wait an hour, then have your blood drawn. (You'll feel either nothing at all from the needle, or a quick sting or pinch.) If your blood sugar level is high, you'll have to come back for a glucose-tolerance test, in which	Your doctor will probably not call you with the result unless the reading is high. A diagnosis of diabetes occurs when any of the following results have been repeated on at least two different days: A fasting blood glucose level that is 126

The Tests	Why You Need It	When and How Often	What to Expect	What the Results Mean
			you'll drink a glucose solution on an empty stomach and have your blood drawn once an hour for 3 hours. The results are usually available within a day.	mg/dL (7.0 mmol/L) or higher. A 2-hour oral glucose tolerance test that is 200 mg/dL (11.1 mmol/L) or higher. Or symptoms of diabetes are present and a random blood glucose test result that is 200 mg/dL (11.1 mmol/L) or higher.
BMI Check (Body Mass Index)	To help maintain a healthy body weight, keep an eye on your BMI.	Annually, beginning at age two.	No side effects unless doing math makes you sick. Or look for a BMI calculator online. BMI = (Weight in Pounds / (Height in inches) x (Height in inches)) x 703.	For adults, body mass index values between 18.5 and 24.9 are considered "normal" or "healthy." BMI values between 25 and 29.9 are considered "overweight" and 30 and above are considered "obese." But since a child's body fat changes as he or she grows over the years, and boys and girls differ in their body fat as they mature, the BMI for children is both age and gender specific. See charts on pages 71–72.

The Tests	Why You Need It	When and How Often	What to Expect	What the Results Mean
Bone Density Test	To determine if you are at risk for osteoporosis, a thinning of the bones, which makes them more prone to breaking. More common in women than in men.	Get tested at menopause if you are at risk for osteoporosis. Otherwise at sixty-five and then every five years. Or as recommended by your health provider.	You will lie on a table fully clothed while an X-ray or CT scanner images your spine, pelvis, lower arm, and thigh. While the procedure itself causes no pain, the technician's manipulation of the body part being examined may cause some discomfort.	If your bone mineral density score is 1 to 2.5 standard deviations below the young adult mean, you have a low bone mass. You will need to take extra calcium and vitamin D daily, according to your doctor's prescription. A score of 2.5 standard deviations or more below the young adult mean indicates the presence of osteoporosis. Your doctor will likely prescribe medication.
Breast Self-Examination (BSE)	To detect a breast cancer, if it exists, early, when it's most likely to be cured. The BSE is an essential part of reducing your risk of breast cancer.	Monthly beginning in the twenties.	Examine yourself several days after the end of your period, when your breasts are least likely to be swollen and tender. Follow the procedure on page 176.	If you feel a lump, make an appointment with your doctor but don't panic. Most women have some lumpy areas in their breasts all the time. And 80 percent of breast lumps that are removed are benign, noncancerous tissue.

The Tests	Why You Need It	When and How Often	What to Expect	What the Results Mean
Chest X-ray	To diagnose lung cancer, tuberculosis, or for a persistent cough, chest pain, coughing up blood, or difficulty breathing. Also for evaluation of the heart and chest wall.	Anytime it's needed, if not then at sixty, or earlier if you are a smoker.	You stand in front of the X-ray machine and must hold your breath when the X-ray is taken. The technician will usually take two views of your lungs. There is no discomfort.	A normal chest X-ray does not necessarily rule out all problems as some cancers are too small or difficult to image. If lung cancer is diagnosed, depending on its progress the doctor will recommend either surgery or chemotherapy.
Cholesterol Test (Lipid Profile)	To track your risk of heart disease. Elevated levels of cholesterol raise your risk of heart attack and stroke.	If you smoke, have diabetes, or have a history of heart disease in the family, check your cholesterol annually by the age of twenty. Otherwise check it every five years until the age of forty-five and annually thereafter.	The cholesterol test is a blood test called a lipid panel or lipid profile. You will need to fast for 9 to 12 hours before the test. The test will measure your total cholesterol, LDL or "bad" cholesterol, HDL or "good" cholesterol, and triglycerides in your blood, measured in milligrams per deciliter of blood (mg/dL).	If your total blood cholesterol level is: Less than 200 mg/dL: Desirable. Between 200–239 mg/dL: Borderline high risk. 240 mg/dL or greater: High risk. If your total cholesterol is high, or if your HDL is less than 40, or your LDL is greater than 130, the doctor may recommend a new diet, an exercise regimen, as well as cholesterol medication.

The Tests	Why You Need It	When and How Often	What to Expect	What the Results Mean
Colonoscopy	To detect colon cancer before symptoms occur by examining colon polyps, tumors, ulcerations, inflammations, pouches, narrowings, or foreign objects within the colon. This is one of three tests for colon cancer, the other two being a Fecal occult blood test (FOBT) and a Sigmoidoscopy, which is similar to a colonoscopy but only covers the lower part of the colon.	Get tested starting at age fifty, then again every five years if at risk, or every ten years if no problems are found.	Your doctor will advise you of the need for a special diet and a very strong laxative prior to the procedure. While under medication to make you drowsy, you will lie on a table while the doctor inserts a long flexible lighted tube with a video camera through the rectum into the colon. The colonoscope also enables the doctor to access the bowel and remove polyps with surgical instruments. If a polyp was removed during the procedure, you may notice a small amount of blood may appear in your bowel movement for a day or so. You may also experience excessive gas pains after the procedure. This also is normal.	If polyps are found they will be removed and biopsied. If cancer is found, you may need surgical treatment or additional testing within three to five years.

The Tests	Why You Need It	When and How Often	What to Expect	What the Results Mean
Dental Checkup	To check teeth and gums for proper development and to deal with any problems discovered.	Every 6 months to a year once adult molars start to come in. Every year as an adult.	Teeth and gums are examined for signs of trouble, plaque is removed from your teeth with a scraper, and teeth are then cleaned and flossed. X-rays are also taken of your teeth to reveal any cavities or other problems.	Any problems can either be taken care of by the dentist or be referred to an oral surgeon, if necessary.
Fetal Occult Blood Test	To detect the presence of blood in the stool, which may be caused by hemorrhoids, anal fissure, colon polyps, colon cancer, and many other conditions that cause bleeding in the gastro-intestinal tract.	Once a year beginning in the fifties.	You will need to avoid certain foods, such as red meat, mushrooms and broccoli, and medicines such as aspirin and antacids two to three days before the test. Your doctor will advise a special diet. The test is usually performed over several days on three different bowel movements to increase the chance of detecting blood in your stool.	A small sample of stool is placed on a chemically treated card with a special solution. If the card turns blue, there is blood in the stool. Not all blood in the stool is caused by cancer. Your doctor will likely suggest further testing, such as a colonoscopy or a sigmoidoscopy.
Flu Vaccine	To greatly reduce the risk of be-coming ill with the flu, a conta-gious respiratory	For all children six to fifty-nine months of age, people who have heart or lung dis-	The "flu shot" is an inactivated vaccine contain-ing killed virus that is given with	About two weeks after vaccination, antibodies de-velop that protect against influenza

The Tests	Why You Need It	When and How Often	What to Expect	What the Results Mean
	illness caused by influenza viruses, which can cause mild to severe illness, even death.	orders or chronic diseases such as diabetes, and people fifty years or older, annually in the fall.	a needle. The nasal-spray flu vaccine is approved for use in healthy people five years to forty-nine years of age who are not pregnant.	virus infection. Flu vaccines will not protect against influenza-like illnesses caused by other viruses.
Group B Streptococcus (GBS) Test in Pregnancy	To check for the presence of GBS bacteria in the vagina.	Between the 35th and 37th weeks of pregnancy.	This test involves swabbing the vagina for surface cells. The cells are placed in a special solution to see if the bacteria grow.	These bacteria, which are found naturally in the vaginas of many women, are the most common cause of blood infections and meningitis in newborns. Pregnant women can transmit GBS to their newborns at birth. The infections are usually treated with antibiotics given intravenously.
Gynecological Exam	To detect and treat GYN conditions early on and prevent them from progressing. Many GYN conditions do not have obvious symptoms.	Beginning when a girl turns eighteen or becomes sexually active, whichever comes first. Then annually, or more frequently if Pap smears are abnormal.	The doctor will examine your breasts for lumps and ask if you have any questions or concerns about your menstrual cycle. Next, you'll rest your feet in the stirrups with your legs spread. The	The cell sample is analyzed to check for cancer or a precancerous condition of the cervix. Results take about a week to get back. If abnormal cells are found, your doctor will recommend further

The Tests	Why You Need It	When and How Often	What to Expect	What the Results Mean
			doctor will then use a speculum to hold the walls of the vagina apart to look inside. The doctor will then insert a swab into your vagina and rub it across your cervix to sample some cells for the Pap smear. The doctor will then remove the speculum and check your ovaries by inserting one or two fingers into your vagina while putting the other hand on your lower abdomen in order to assess the size, shape, and position of your uterus, ovaries, and fallopian tubes and check for swelling or growths.	testing to confirm the result and eventually perhaps a biopsy.
Hearing and Vision Tests	To detect any hearing or vision problems as early as possible.	At 6–9 months, 18–24 months, 3–3.5 years, and around the time a child starts primary school. Every three years for teenagers.	Hearing tests: In newborns, a painless clicking sound is played though a tiny earpiece placed in the baby's outer ear. A computer	If hearing or vision problems are detected, a doctor can treat the problem, perhaps with glasses or a hearing aid, and provide ac-

The Tests	Why You Need It	When and How Often	What to Expect	What the Results Mean
		Then as needed, or every two years for hearing beginning at age fifty and vision after age forty-five.	records the reaction sounds that should take place in the ear's cochlea. It is painless and can be done while the baby is asleep. Older children and adults are asked to raise their hand or press a button as tones or words are played through headphones, earplugs, or a bone conductor. Vision Tests: A newborn's eyes are examined for any physical defects, including redness, cross-eyes, and cloudiness. Later, vision tests involve reading letters from a certain distance away.	cess to special support services, if needed.
Hormone Check	To check on the loss of estrogen and progesterone hormones as well as thyroid hormones at menopause.	At menopause.	Medication in pill form, if hormone therapy is right for you	Your doctor will offer a treatment plan if your estrogen, progesterone, or thyroid levels are significantly reduced.

The Tests	Why You Need It	When and How Often	What to Expect	What the Results Mean
Mammogram	To detect breast cancer early, when it's most curable. Many times a mammogram can pick up a tumor before it is felt.	If you're at high risk for breast cancer, you should get your first mammogram (called a baseline mammogram) in your thirties, then annually, or earlier if you have a first degree relative with breast cancer. Otherwise annually beginning at age forty.	A technician will position and compress each breast between two plates so that a special camera can take clear X-ray images of each breast. The procedure is mildly uncomfortable for most women, but pain-ful for a few. Mammography today involves only a tiny amount of radiation—even less than a standard chest X-ray.	The baseline mammogram is used for comparison to subsequent mammograms to see if any changes have taken place in the breasts. If a mass is spotted in the breast, the doctor may recommend an ultrasound or MRI to confirm if it is indeed a solid mass, in which case a biopsy may be necessary.
Mental Health Screening	To determine if you are clinically depressed and require treatment.	As needed. For example, if you're feeling "down," sad, or hopeless, and have little interest in doing anything for a period of two weeks or more, have your doctor test you for depression. Don't wait to see the doctor, as the longer you wait, the harder depression is to treat.	You will be asked to respond to a number of questions by answering "yes" or "no" based on how you felt during the previous week. Your answers will allow the doctor to determine if depression or some other mental health problem such as bipolar disorder, generalized anxiety disorder, or post-traumatic stress disorder is involved.	If the doctor finds you depressed, treatment will consist of counseling, medicine, or both. Treatment takes several weeks. Contrary to popular belief, mental health problems are treatable.

The Tests	Why You Need It	When and How Often	What to Expect	What the Results Mean
Non-stress Test	For pregnant women, to check if the baby is responding normally to a stimulus.	If the baby is past due, the test is taken one week after the due date. Also performed in high risk pregnancies, or when fetal movement is uncertain, anytime after the 26th to 28th week.	You may be asked to eat something just before the test in an effort to stimulate your baby to move around. For the next hour you will be lying down strapped to one monitor that tracks your baby's heartbeat and movement and another that records the contractions in your uterus. A technician will listen to and watch your baby's heartbeat and movements on screen. You may be asked to press a button when you feel the baby move. If your baby doesn't move, he may be asleep, and a buzzer may be used to wake him.	The result is considered normal, and your baby "reactive," if your baby's heart beats faster while he's moving for at least 15 seconds on two separate occasions during a 20-minute period. A nonreactive result could indicate that your baby isn't getting enough oxygen or a problem with the placenta and your doctor may decide to do a biophysical profile.

The Tests	Why You Need It	When and How Often	What to Expect	What the Results Mean
Pap Smear	To check for treatable health problems such as STDs or cervical cancer.	Beginning at eighteen (or younger, if sexually active), then every two–three years.	The doctor will use what looks like a cotton swab to gently scrape the inside of your cervix. It usually does not hurt at all, though some women report feeling a brief little twinge.	If a sexually transmitted disease (STD) or cervical cancer is found, treatment is begun.
Physical Examination (Adult)	To screen for diseases, assess risk of future medical problems, encourage healthy lifestyle, and maintain relationship with a doctor in case of illness.	Every three–five years until the age of fifty, then annually.	You will strip down to your underwear. First weight, temperature, pulse and blood pressure are measured. Then the main organs are examined. If a particular disease is suspected, specific tests are conducted.	The "physical" is the cornerstone of preventive medicine and the data collected becomes a part of the person's medical record. If any problem is discovered, a diagnosis is made and a treatment plan devised.
Physical Examination (Children)	To check if the child is growing and developing normally. Also gives parents a chance to talk with the doctor about any issues that arise, to resolve them, and keep the child healthy.	Annually until the teens then every couple of years.	The doctor will listen to the heart and lungs with a stethoscope, look in the ears, nose and throat, examine the eyes, check reflexes with a rubber hammer, feel the abdomen, perform a genital exam, and check that	The results go into a chart that will be used to follow the child's growth and development. Any negative test, or signs of problems, will be assessed with further tests before any treatment is begun.

The Tests	Why You Need It	When and How Often	What to Expect	What the Results Mean
			the spine is not crooked. Weight and height, blood pressure and temperature will be taken as well. Hearing and vision may also be checked.	
Physical (Prenatal)	To find and treat any health problems that can affect the baby's health. To get to know the person who will be directly involved in your care during labor and delivery.	First visit once you're pregnant.	You will be asked about your family's health history. Blood is drawn and urine taken for lab work. Your heart, lungs and thyroid function are assessed. The abdomen and pelvis are examined, and the height of the uterus is measured.	Indicates the overall health of the mother-to-be. Provides mother's blood type and Rh factor. Urine is tested for infections or diabetes. Provides your baby's due date and a reference point for future visits when the baby's growth is assessed.
Pneumococcal vaccine	For prevention of the pneumococcal disease because the treatment of this infection has become more difficult as the disease has become more resistant to such drugs as penicillin.	At age sixty-five, then every five to ten years.	Half of those who get the vaccine have very mild side effects, a redness or pain where the shot is given. Few develop a fever, or muscle aches. Severe allergic reactions are very rare.	The vaccine usually protects against twenty-three types of pneumococcal bacteria within two to three weeks of getting the shot. The very young, very old, or very sick might not respond well or at all to the vaccination.

The Tests	Why You Need It	When and How Often	What to Expect	What the Results Mean
Prenatal Checkups	To track the health of the mother and the baby.	Once a month until your 28th week; every two weeks from the 28th to the 34th week; then weekly after the 34th week.	Prenatal visits are usually shorter than the initial visit for the full physical. You will be asked for a urine sample to check for sugar, protein, and signs of infection. Your blood pressure will be taken, the height of the uterus will be measured, and the mother's weight will be recorded. Toward the end of the pregnancy, the doctor will check the baby's positioning by feeling around your abdomen.	A woman should gain 10 to 12 pounds during the first half of her pregnancy and 15 to 17 during the second half. Sugar in urine indicates gestational diabetes while protein in the urine or a sudden rise in blood pressure may indicate complications during pregnancy.
Prostate Cancer Screening	To detect prostate cancer in men.	Annually beginning at fifty.	As part of a routine physical exam, the doctor will insert a finger in the anus and feel through the rectal wall for any enlargement of the prostate. It's uncomfortable but not usually painful. The doctor will also do a prostate specific antigen	The normal range for the PSA test is less than 4.0 nanograms per milliliter (ng/mL). But PSA levels are elevated not only in prostate cancer, but in an enlargement of the prostate called Benign Prostatic Hyperplasia as well, so it's not a definitive test.

The Tests	Why You Need It	When and How Often	What to Expect	What the Results Mean
			(PSA) test, a blood test that can be helpful to detect prostate cancer. To prepare for a PSA, avoid having sex 24 hours prior; you may also have to skp medications before the test.	If prostate cancer is confirmed, treatment may involve surgery, radiation therapy or hormone therapy, depending on the size of the tumor, whether it has spread to other parts of your body, and your overall health.
Skin Exam (Mole Screening)	To avoid skin cancer and other serious skin problems.	Do a monthly self-test and have an annual skin check by a doctor beginning in your thirties. Earlier if you are at high risk for skin cancer.	Self Test: Stand in front of a full-length mirror. Check every inch of your skin, including the bottoms of your feet. Use a hand-held mirror to check your back. Have someone help you check the top of your head, using a blow-dryer if necessary to move your hair out of the way. The dermatologist will examine your body from head to toe and may measure or image any unusual moles.	If you notice a new mole that doesn't look like your other moles, or a mole that has changed its appearance, see your doctor. The dermatologist will take samples from suspicious looking moles. Skin cancer can be treated successfully if it's treated early.

The Tests	Why You Need It	When and How Often	What to Expect	What the Results Mean
STD Tests	To detect and treat Sexually Transmitted Diseases, which can cause cancer, liver disease, pelvic inflammatory disease, infertility, pregnancy problems, and other complications and life-threatening diseases.	Beginning when a person becomes sexually active. Any time you start a new sexual relationship and frequently in non-monogamous relationships.	Begins with a genital examination. For women, the examination is similar to having a Pap smear. The doctor will take swabs for chlamydia and gonorrhea from the cervix, and swabs from the vaginal walls for yeast, bacterial vaginosis, and trichomoniasis. For men, the doctor will check the lymph nodes in the groin as well as feel the testicles for lumps or discomfort. In the gonorrhea test, which is uncomfortable but brief, the doctor will insert a thin swab a short distance into the urethra and gently rotate it to collect any organisms. For chlamydia, a urine sample is collected. For both men and women,	If tested positive for an STD, medications will be prescribed. For STDs that can't be cured, like herpes, treatment aims at relieving the symptoms.

The Tests	Why You Need It	When and How Often	What to Expect	What the Results Mean
			HIV, syphilis, and hepatitis are tested through blood tests.	
Tetanus Booster	To help the body make antibodies to fight infections that occur from skin wounds that become contaminated by a bacterium that causes lockjaw. Not just for puncture wounds; cracks in the skin can become infected while working in the garden, for example.	Recommended every five to ten years, throughout life. A person who gets a deep puncture wound more than five years after the last tetanus booster may be advised to get another one.	A tetanus booster is a shot given after the first series of vaccinations. Usually it is combined with the diphtheria booster. The combination is called a Td booster. Few people have problems with the vaccine; side effects, if any, are usually mild.	Better to prevent lockjaw with the booster than to have to treat the disease.
Thyroid test (TSH)	To screen adults for thyroid disorders, screen newborns for an underactive thyroid, monitor thyroid replacement therapy, and diagnose and monitor female infertility problems.	Every five years starting at the age of thirty-five.	No special preparation needed. Blood is drawn from a vein, usually from the inside of the elbow or the back of the hand.	A high Thyroid Stimulating Hormone (TSH) result often means an underactive thyroid gland, while a low TSH result can indicate an overactive thyroid gland (hyperthyroidism). In either case your doctor will prescribe the appropriate medication.

The Tests	Why You Need It	When and How Often	What to Expect	What the Results Mean
Triple Screen Test (Alpha Foetal Protein 3 or 4)	For pregnant women, to check the levels of protein and hormones being produced by the fetus.	Between the 15th and 20th weeks of pregnancy.	Your blood will be drawn and you will be weighed and asked when your last period began or what your expected due date is. The results of the blood test, which depends on your weight and stage of pregnancy, are available within two to three days.	Enables doctors to identify pregnancies that are at a higher risk for brain and spinal cord birth defects as well as genetic ab-normalities. If a problem shows up, additional tests may be needed.
Ultrasound	For pregnant women, to deter-mine the health of the baby, its position, and due date. It's also use-ful for identifying multiple preg-nancies, some birth defects, and sometimes the sex of the baby.	Usually per-formed at eigh-teen to twenty weeks. Can be repeated, depend-ing on the need.	Early in the preg-nancy, a full blad-der is required so you will be asked to drink a lot of water and not urinate. While lying down, your lower abdomen will be coated with a clear jelly so that a sensor that looks like a microphone will be able to slide around easily against your skin. As the techni-cian moves the sensor back and forth over your abdomen, a video image of the fetus appears on	The results tell you whether or not the baby is growing nor-mally. Some re-sults are available immediately, but a full evaluation may take a week. If the baby's geni-tals are visible— and you want to know your baby's gender—you can find out at this time.

The Tests	Why You Need It	When and How Often	What to Expect	What the Results Mean
			the monitor. Its heartbeat, arms and legs, and internal organs may be visible.	
Vaccines (Childhood)	To protect your child from some of the deadliest diseases in history.	For most of these vaccines, the first shots should be given when children are still babies. See chart on page 35 for complete timetable of all the vaccines.	Vaccines are very safe, but like any other medicine they can occasionally cause reactions. After immunization, children may be fussy due to fever, aches, or other mild reactions. Serious reactions are rare.	Vaccines give the immune system just enough knowledge of a potential invader for the body to produce the antibodies it needs should the real virus ever attack—and the vaccine does so without getting you sick.

Sources and Resources

We have many sources of health and medical information available to us today. Some of the best and most up-to-date material can be found on the Internet, though not everything you find online is reliable. I recommend the following sites if you would like to get more information on the topics discussed in this book. Of course, you can visit my site as well:

Ask Dr. Manny
http://www.askdrmanny.com/

Alzheimer's Foundation of
America
http://alzfdn.org/

American Academy of
Dermatology
http://www.aad.org/

American Cancer Society
http://www.cancer.org/

American Diabetes Association
http://www.diabetes.org/

American Lung Association
www.lungus.org/

American Obesity Association
http://www.obesity.org/

American Psychiatric Association
http://www.psych.org/

American Stroke Association
http://www.strokeassociation.org/

Baby Center
http://www.babycenter.com/

Better Hearing Institute
http://betterhearing.org/

Centers for Disease Control
http://www.cdc.gov/

Cleveland Clinic
http://www.clevelandclinic.org/

Cool Nurse
http://www.coolnurse.com/

eNotes Health
http://health.enotes.com/

EyeMDLink
http://www.eyemdlink.com/

FamilyDoctor
http://familydoctor.org/

Fox News Health
http://www.foxnews.com/health

Hackensack University
Medical Center
http://www.humed.com/
humc_ency/

Health Forums
https://www.healthforums.com/

HealthLink Medical College of
Wisconsin
http://healthlink.mcw.edu/

Health Square
http://www.healthsquare.com/

Health Status: Internet
Assessments
http://www.healthstatus.com/

KidsHealth
http://kidshealth.org/

Mayo Clinic
http://www.mayoclinic.com/

MedicineNet
http://www.medicinenet.com/

Medline Plus
http://medlineplus.gov/

MSN Health & Fitness
http://health.msn.com/

National Institutes of Health
http://health.nih.gov/

National Mental Health
Association
http://www.nmha.org/

National Osteoporosis Foundation
http://nof.org/

National Sleep Foundation
http://www.sleepfoundation.org/

Net Doctor
http://www.netdoctor.co.uk/

RealAge
http://www.realage.com/

The Health Check
http://www.thehealthcheck.com

The Site Health & Wellbeing
http://www.thesite.org/
healthandwellbeing/generalhealth

U.S. Food and Drug
Administration
http://www.fda.gov/

Vital Select
http://www.vitalselect.com

Vitamins Solutions
http://www.vitaminssolutions.com

Index

bone density test, 284
Botox treatments, 218
bowel cancer, 125
brachial plexus, 11
breast cancer, 21, 173–78, 237, 242, 251,
    252
    birth control pills and, 108, 174
    in men, 178
    prevention of, 174–75
    reconstructive surgery after, 177,
        217
    risk factors of, 108, 174, 196, 242
    screenings for, 175, 176, 189, 221, 222,
        257, 291
    self-examining for, 96, 129, 162, 175,
        176, 178, 190, 222, 277, 284–85
    stages of, 177
    treatments for, 177–78
breast-feeding, 21, 26–27, 39, 106,
    174
breast implants, 116, 218–19
breast/ovarian cancer syndrome, 227
breast reduction, 217
British Medical Journal, 225
bronchitis, 4, 34, 109, 111
bronchodilator, 61
bronchoscopy, 238, 239
bulimia, 76–78, 241
burns, prevention of, 31

caffeine, 149, 195
C. albicans, 148
calcitonin, 242
calcium, 138, 149, 195, 234, 255
    in children, 28
    osteoporosis and, 241, 242, 243, 284
calcium stones, 146–47
calories:
    burned per minute in activities, 169
    intake vs. burning of, 134, 136, 166–67,
        213
camps, obesity, 69
cancer, 74, 89, 109, 134, 150, 167, 179, 186,
    221, 252, 285, 287
    tests for, 91, 96
    see also specific types of cancer
car accidents, 86
carbohydrates, 10, 134, 135, 181
    refined, 66, 125, 198
    simple, 83
carbon monoxide poisoning, 31
carcino-embryonic antigen (CEA), 254
cardiocatheterization, 228

cardiovascular disease, 75, 195, 213, 215,
    234, 274
    see also heart disease
carotid endarterectomy, 235
cataracts, 249–50
CAT scans, 125, 139, 228, 238, 254, 273
cavities, 76
celery, 137
cerebral palsy, 12, 13
cervical cancer, 91, 96, 109, 151, 288–89,
    293, 297
cervical cap, 105
cesarean section (C section), 14, 15
chemical peels, 218
chemotherapy, 22, 147, 151, 160, 177, 208,
    210, 237, 238, 240, 252, 254, 274, 285
chenodeoxycholic, 202
chest X-rays, 238, 257, 285
chickenpox, 13, 35
chicken soup, 37
childhood leukemia, 22
Child Magazine, 73
childproofing, of home, 30–33
Chinese, 197
chlamydia, 89–90, 105, 297
choking, prevention of, 33
cholecystectomy, 202, 239
cholelithiasis, 201–3
cholesterol, xvii, 65*n*, 188, 214, 228, 229,
    231, 234
    testing of, 129, 162, 190, 222, 257, 277,
        285
cholesterol stones, 201, 203
chondroitin, 155
chorionic villus sampling (CVS), 6
chronic gingivitis, 76
chronic hypertension, 8
chronic lymphocytic leukemia (CLL),
    207, 208
chronic myelogenous leukemia (CML),
    207
chronic obstructive pulmonary disease
    (COPD), 111
Cialis, 173
circumcision, 24–25
Claritin, 59
clean catch, 145
Clomiphene, 199
Clonidine, 49, 195
cobranding, 68–69
coenzyme Q10, 212
Cognex, 270–71
Coil, 107

colds, common, 36–38, 42
  remedies for, 37, 38
  symptoms of, 59
colitis, 123
collagen injections, 218
colon cancer, 125, 237, 251, 252, 253–55,
    272
  calcium supplements and, 138
  prevention of, 254
  symptoms of, 253–54
  tests for, 222, 254, 257, 277, 286
colonoscopies, 125, 221, 222, 254, 257,
    277, 286, 287
colorectal cancer tests, 222, 257, 277
community-acquired pneumonia, 275
computer-intense lifestyle, 101–3
Concerta, 49
condoms, 105
conductive hearing loss, 245
congenital glaucoma, 248
conjunctivitis (pinkeye), 39–40
Connecticut, 73
constipation, 125, 126–28, 144, 254, 273
contact dermatitis, 112
contraception, 104–8
contraceptive ring, 106
convulsions, 34
cord blood, umbilical, 21–23
corn syrup, 65
coronary artery disease, 104, 227–29, 230,
    231, 263
  see also heart disease
corticosteroids, 9, 118
cosmetic surgery, see plastic surgery
Coxsackie, 40
Crohn's disease, 123, 124–26, 253
croup, 34
cryosurgery, 151
CT scanners, 231, 284
cuts, prevention of, 33
Cylert, 49
cystic fibrosis, 4, 5
cysts, 62
cytomegalovirus (CMV), 13, 95

dating ultrasound, 6
Davis, Nancy, 161
deafness, 12, 45
  see also hearing loss
de-bulking procedure, 273–74
decongestants, 37
dehydration, 122, 123, 124, 125, 147
dementia, 269, 270

Demerol, 4
demyelination, 159
dental health, 54, 74–76, 97, 129, 162, 189,
    190, 222, 257, 277, 287
  in Eighth Decade, 266, 268
Depo Provera, 107
depression, 48, 53, 79, 85, 110, 138, 149,
    170, 179, 180, 185, 197, 198, 210, 220,
    236, 257, 266, 271
  in adolescents, 79–84, 86
  bulimia and, 78
  diet and, 82–83
  manic, see bipolar disorder
  myths about, 84
  postpartum, 23
  screenings for, 129, 162, 190, 222, 291
  signs of, 80
  treatment of, 81–82, 83, 181–82
Dexedrine, 49
diabetes, 148, 153, 156, 173, 184, 212–16,
    263, 271, 274, 285, 288
  damage caused by, 11, 74, 75, 214, 231,
    233, 234, 245, 246–47, 248, 249, 252
  juvenile (Type 1), 23, 74, 75, 213, 215,
    216
  monitoring of, 214–15, 222, 282–83
  obesity and, 64, 212, 213–14
  in pregnancy, 3, 8, 10–11, 69–70, 214,
    282, 294, 295
  Type 2, 74, 212–16
Diagnostic and Statistical Manual (DSM),
    180
diaper rash, 52
diaphragm, 105
diarrhea, 122–24, 125, 149, 253–54, 273
diastolic pressure, 186
diet, 125, 128, 156, 161, 187, 215, 216, 218,
    229, 271, 276, 279, 287
  andropause and, 198, 199
  artificial sweeteners in, 167–68
  calorie intake vs. calories burned in,
    134, 136, 166–67, 213–14
  colon cancer and, 253, 254–55
  in Eighth Decade, 266–67
  in Fifth Decade, 165–68
  in Fourth Decade, 135–37
  gallbladder cancer prevention with, 240
  gastrointestinal disorders and, 124,
    126–27, 128
  high-fiber, 127, 128
  hypertension and, 187, 188
  kidney stones and, 146–47
  lupus and, 117

macular degeneration and, 265, 266
meal scheduling and, 136–37
menopause and, 195, 196–97
mental health and, 82–83, 181–82
metabolism and, 136–37, 199–200
osteoporosis and, 241, 243
ovarian cancer and, 272
PMS and, 149
processed foods in, 64–66, 135
skin health and, 142
stroke prevention and, 234
vision problems prevention with, 250
see also obesity
diffuse toxic goiter, 143
dilation, 14–15
dopamine, 210–12
Down's syndrome, 4
prenatal tests for, 6, 281
drowning, prevention of, 32
drug-induced lupus, 116
drugs, recreational, 85, 88, 101, 115, 128,
133, 162, 170, 185, 234
drusen, 264
"dry" AMD, 264
dry-eye syndrome, 249
dysmenorrhea, 148–49, 172
dyspareunia, 171

ear infections, 38–39, 40
eating disorders, 53, 76–79, 241
echinacea, 37
E. coli, 122
eczema, 111–12
Eighth Decade (ages 70–100), 259–77
Alzheimer's disease in, 269–71
dental care in, 266, 268
diet in, 266–67
home injuries in, 276
macular degeneration in, 263–66
medications in, 267–68
ovarian cancer in, 271–74
percent of function in, 262–63
pneumonia in, 274–76
tests and vaccines in, 275, 277
electric shock, prevention of, 32
electrocardiogram (ECG or EKG), 228,
229
embolic strokes, 233
embolization, 151
emphysema, 4, 109, 111, 274
endometriosis, 125, 149–50, 152, 172
endoscopy, 122
environmental hormones, 199–200

epilepsy, 13
Epstein-Barr virus (EBV), 95
Equal, 167
erectile dysfunction (E.D.), 170, 172–73
esophageal cancer, 120
essential hypertension, 186
estrogen, 62n, 104, 106, 108, 171, 178, 198,
200, 239, 241, 290
and menopause, 193–97
natural, 196–97
eustachian tubes, 38–39
exercise, 73, 75, 104, 115, 117, 127, 128,
136, 147, 149, 161, 165, 172, 174, 187,
188, 195, 199, 212, 215, 216, 229, 234,
242, 243, 255, 279
arthritis and, 156, 157
drinking water during, 168–69
in Fifth Decade, 168–69
mental health and, 82, 126, 183, 185
metabolism boosted by, 168, 200, 267
obesity and lack of, 67–69
sports injuries due to, 156
eye exams, 188

face-lifts, 219–20
fats, 135
saturated, 65n, 66, 234
unsaturated, 136
fatty acids, 135, 181
Fecal occult blood test (FORT), 222, 257,
277, 286, 287
ferrous iron, 212
fetal alcohol syndrome, 4
fever, 37, 42, 123, 145, 300
rheumatic, 41
fibroids, uterine, 150–51, 172
fibromyalgia, 125, 158
Fifth Decade (ages 40–49), 163–90
breast cancer and, 173–78
diet plan in, 165–68
exercise in, 168–69
hypertension in, 185–88
mental health in, 179–84
sexual problems in, 169–73
stress in, 184–85
tests and vaccines in, 188–89, 190
fifth disease, 13, 40–41
fifties, *see* Sixth Decade
First Decade (ages 0–9), 17–54
ADD/ADHD in, 47–50
autism diagnosis in, 43–47
avoiding food allergies in, 27–29
childproofing of home in, 30–33

Rhinocort, 59
rhinoplasty, 217
rhinoviruses, 36
rickets, 65
"ringing ears," 245, 246
Ritalin, 49
Robitussin, 268
Roizen, Michael F., xiii–xiv
rosacea, 114–15
rotavirus, 122
rubella (German measles), 5, 13, 35

saline breast implants, 218
salmon, 142
salmonella, 122
sarcoidosis, 118–20, 147
saturated fats, 65n, 66, 234
saw palmetto, 139, 206
scarlet fever, 41
schizophrenia, 180, 211
seasonal allergies, 29, 30, 57–59, 60
secondary hypertension, 186
Second Decade (ages 10–19), 55–97
    acne in, 61–64
    asthma in, 60–61
    dental health in, 74–76
    depression in, 53, 79–84, 85, 86
    eating disorders in, 53, 76–79
    obesity in, 53, 57, 64–74, 154
    seasonal allergies in, 57–59
    STDs acquired in, 88–94
    tests and vaccines in, 97, 293–94
    see also adolescence
selenium, 206, 255
self-esteem, 54, 80, 85, 87
sensorineural hearing loss, 245–46
Seventh Decade (ages 60–69), 223–57
    colon cancer in, 253–55
    gallbladder cancer in, 239–40
    hearing loss in, 244–47
    heart disease in, 227–30
    lung cancer in, 237–39
    osteoporosis in, 240–43
    pancreatic cancer in, 251–52
    strokes in, 232–36
    tests and vaccines in, 257
    vision problems in, 247–51
seventies, see Eighth Decade
sex, 145
    in adolescence, 85, 87, 88–94
    contraception and, 104–8
    physical issues in, 169–73, 204, 205,
      206, 210, 235

during pregnancy, 7–8
    unprotected, 85
sexual abuse, 80, 82, 171
sexually transmitted diseases (STDs), xv,
    7, 88–94, 107, 293
    circumcision and, 24
    prevention of, 94, 105, 106
    tests for, 91, 96, 97, 129, 162, 189, 190,
      293, 297–98
Shell Oil, 225
sickle cell anemia, 5
sigmoidoscopy, 286, 287
silicone breast implants, 116, 218
simple carbohydrates, 83
site-specific ovarian cancer syndrome,
    272
Sixth Decade (ages 50–59), 191–222
    andropause in, 197–99
    diabetes in, 212–16
    gallstones in, 201–3
    healthy metabolism in, 199–200
    leukemia and, 207–8
    menopause in, 193–97, 199
    non-Hodgkin's lymphoma and, 209–10
    Parkinson's disease in, 210–12
    plastic surgery in, 216–20
    prostate health in, 203–6
    tests and vaccines in, 221, 222
sixties, see Seventh Decade
skin, 165
    cancer of, 139–42, 204, 296
    improving appearance of, 142
    problems affecting, 111–15, 128
    screenings, 97, 129, 141–42, 162,
      188–89, 190, 222, 257, 277, 296
slapped-cheek syndrome, 13, 40–41
sleeping problems, 101, 102–3
    in menopause, 194
smoking, 26, 39, 75, 104, 106, 121, 128,
    133, 142, 162, 173, 184, 185, 229, 279
    in adolescence, 57, 85, 86–88
    asthma and, 60, 109
    health risks of, 4, 109, 111, 115, 187,
      188, 195, 206, 228, 234, 240, 241, 243,
      249, 252, 266, 285
    lung cancer and, 4, 87, 88, 111, 237, 238
    pregnancy and, 4, 109
    quitting of, 109–11
snacks, healthy, 137
sodium, 187
soft drinks, 137
sore throats, 41
South America, 167

South Beach Diet, 165–66
spermicidal cream, 105–6
spermicide, 106
sphygmomanometer, 282
spina bifida, 5, 214
Splenda, 167
sponge, 105–6
sports injuries, 156
squamous cell carcinoma, 237
stem cells, 212
sterilization, 107–8
steroids, 12, 61, 113, 117–18, 160, 241, 249
stevia, 167–68
strangulation, prevention of, 32
Strattera, 49
strep throat, 41, 113
stress, 63, 85, 87, 113, 116, 120, 126, 152, 170, 172, 199, 234
    bipolar disorder and avoiding of, 183–84
    in Fifth Decade, 184–85
    hormonal imbalances due to, 200
    hypertension link to, 187–88
    post-traumatic, 184–85, 291
    pregnancy and, 9, 12
    repetitive, 102
    signs of, 185
strokes, 64, 66, 106, 127, 186, 188, 196, 213, 214, 215, 231, 232–36, 248, 271
    coping with, 235–36
    preventive measures for, 234
    risk factors for, 233–34
    symptoms of, 232–33
    treatment of, 234–35
substance abuse, 84–86, 181
    warning signs of, 86
    see also alcohol; smoking
sudden infant death syndrome (SIDS), 26–27
sugars, 135
suicide, 63, 84
    adolescents and, 49–50, 79, 84, 85
sunburns, 64
sun exposure, 113, 120, 140–41
sun poisoning, 116
sunscreen, 140, 141
sweeteners, artificial, 116, 167–68
syphilis, 24, 89, 91, 105, 298
systolic pressure, 186

talcum powder, 272
tamoxifen, 175, 178
targeted ultrasounds, 7

Tay-Sachs, 5
T cells, 113
tear film, 249
teenagers, see adolescence; Second Decade
television:
    advertising on, 68–69
    viewing of, 68
terbutaline sulfate, 12
teriparatide, 242
testicular torsion, 52
testosterone, 170, 193, 200, 241
    andropause and, 197–99
tests:
    in First Decade, 19, 54
    in Second Decade, 97
    in Third Decade, 129
    in Fourth Decade, 162
    in Fifth Decade, 188–89, 190
    in Sixth Decade, 221, 222
    in Seventh Decade, 257
    in Eighth Decade, 277
    master checklist for, 281–300
    for newborns, 19, 20, 54, 289–90
    prenatal, 5–7, 11, 16, 153, 281, 288, 292, 294, 295, 299
tetanus booster, 35, 97, 129, 162, 190, 222, 257, 298
thimerosal, 35
Third Decade (ages 20–29), xvii, 99–129
    autoimmune diseases and, 115–20
    computer-intense lifestyle of, 101–3
    contraception and, 104–8
    gastrointestinal disorders in, 120–28
    migraine headaches in, 103–4
    quitting smoking in, 109–11
    skin conditions in, 111–15, 128
    tests and vaccines in, 129
thirties, see Fourth Decade
thrombolytic drugs, 235
thrombotic strokes, 233
thyroid, 142–44, 147, 245
    disease of, 127, 298
thyroiditis, 143
thyroid tests (TSH), 143, 298
tinnitus, 246
toddlers, 52, 54
    autism in, 43–45
    childproofing for, 30–33
    see also First Decade
tooth decay, 268
Townshend, Pete, 280
toxic shock syndrome, 105

women (*cont.*)
  gynecological exams of, 96, 97, 129,
    162, 189, 190, 222, 257, 277, 288–89
  gynecological problems in, 148–51
  hormone replace therapy for, 143, 174,
    195, 196, 234, 242, 290
  infertility in, 152–53
  menopause in, 151, 171, 174, 193–97,
    199, 222, 241, 249, 272, 284, 290
  osteoporosis in, 240, 284
  ovarian cancer in, 271–74
  sexual issues in, 170–72

  urinary tract infections in, 144–46
  see also pregnancy
Women's Health Initiative (WHI), 196

yeast infections, 51–52, 148, 171
YOU: The Owners Manual (Roizen and
  Oz), xiii

zeaxanthin, 265
zinc, 37
Zoloft, 195
Zyrtec, 59